THE FIRST YEAR™

HIV

An Essential Guide for the Newly Diagnosed

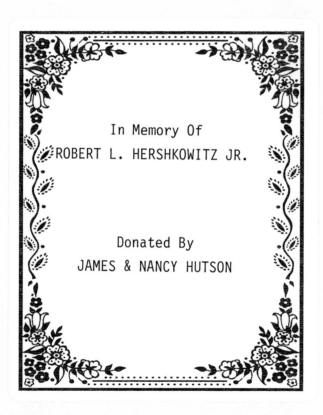

In Memory Of
ROBERT L. HERSHKOWITZ JR.

Donated By
JAMES & NANCY HUTSON

BRETT GRODECK is an online editor for the Rand Corporation, a nonprofit think tank. He has been HIV-positive for fifteen years. An accomplished writer, his articles have appeared in the *Chicago Reader, Chicago* magazine, *Men's Fitness,* and various HIV treatment journals. As a patient advocate, he has consulted for the Food and Drug Administration's antiviral advisory committee. Grodeck lives in Santa Monica, California.

THE COMPLETE FIRST YEAR™ SERIES

THE FIRST YEAR™

HIV

An Essential Guide for the Newly Diagnosed

Brett Grodeck

Foreword by Daniel S. Berger, M.D.

MARLOWE & COMPANY ■ NEW YORK

THE FIRST YEAR™—HIV:
An Essential Guide for the Newly Diagnosed
Copyright © 2003 by Brett Grodeck
Foreword copyright © 2003 by Daniel S. Berger, M.D.
Copyright © 2003 by Tanya Maiboroda for illustrations
appearing on pages 37–38 and 104

Published by
Marlowe & Company
An Imprint of Avalon Publishing Group Incorporated
161 William Street, 16th Floor
New York, NY 10038

The First Year™ and A Patient-Expert Walks You Through
Everything You Need to Learn and Do™ are trademarks of
the Avalon Publishing Group.

Library of Congress Cataloging-in-Publication Data
Godeck, Brett.
    The first year—HIV : an essential guide for the newly
diagnosed / by Brett Grodeck.
        p. cm.
Includes bibliographical references and index.
    ISBN 1-56924-490-1
    1. HIV infections—Popular works. I. Title: HIV.
II. Title.
RC606.64.G765 2003
362.1'969792—dc21   2003041270

ISBN 13: 978-1-56924-490-6

9   8   7   6   5

*Designed by Pauline Neuwirth,
    Neuwirth and Associates, Inc.*

Printed in the United States of America

Distributed by Publishers Group West

Contents

FOREWORD BY DANIEL S. BERGER, M.D.   xi

INTRODUCTION   xv

DAY 1
Living: HIV Is Manageable   1
Learning: Adjusting to the News   4

DAY 2
Living: Emotional Overload   7
Learning: Be Careful Whom You Tell   11

DAY 3
Living: A Few Simple Facts   14
Learning: Healthy Thinking   17

DAY 4
Living: Stigma and Shame   20
Learning: Spirituality and Religion   23

DAY 5
Living: Free Services Are Available   28
Learning: Frequently Asked Questions   31

DAY 6
Living: Consider a Support Group   34
Learning: Needles   36

DAY 7
Living: Tracking Your Health   39
Learning: Take Your Time to Adjust   47

FIRST-WEEK MILESTONE   51

WEEK 2
Living: Finding the Best HIV Doctor   53
Learning: The Virus Versus You   61

WEEK 3
Living: Dealing with People: Disclosing the News   65
Learning: Urban Legends, Myths, and Anti-AIDS Propaganda   71

WEEK 4
Living: Alternative Medicine: Mind Over Money?   76
Learning: T-Cell Counts and Viral Load Tests   84

FIRST-MONTH MILESTONE   91

MONTH 2
Living: Dating and Sex   93
Learning: Herpes and HPV   106

MONTH 3
Living: Anxiety, Depression, and Suicide   116
Learning: Fixing the Funk: Treating Anxiety and Depression   124

MONTH 4
Living: Substance Abuse   132
Learning: Fixing the Addiction   142

MONTH 5
Living: Nutrition and Exercise   151
Learning: Why and When to Treat HIV   166

MONTH 6
Living: Getting Healthcare   175
Learning: Discrimination at Work   186

HALF-YEAR MILESTONE 197

MONTH 7
Living: The Game Plan for HIV Treatment 199
Learning: Meet the Drug Families 211

MONTH 8
Living: Viral Hepatitis 215
Learning: Treating Hepatitis 221

MONTH 9
Living: Long-Term Effects of Treatment 225
Learning: Strategies to Combat Body Shape Changes 230

MONTH 10
Living: Taking Pills Every Day 234
Learning: Managing Short-Term Side Effects 238

MONTH 11
Living: Planning for Plan B 244
Learning: If Treatment Fails 249

MONTH 12
Living: Having Children 256
Learning: Keep Moving Forward 261

GLOSSARY 267

BIBLIOGRAPHY 271

RESOURCES 283

ACKNOWLEDGMENTS 309

INDEX 311

Foreword

by Daniel S. Berger, M.D.

THERE ISN'T a day that goes by that I don't reflect on the struggles of the early years of the AIDS epidemic. In some ways those times have passed, but they have left a deep impression on me and on many others who lived through that bleak period of AIDS history. We had to learn many hard lessons and maneuver around many obstacles to get where we are today, but the wisdom and experience we gained have contributed to our deeper understanding of what individuals can do to reach a better "sense of well-being" and fitness. As you read through this book it will become obvious that different factors all play important roles in maintaining your health in HIV-infection. Factors that were previously considered outside the mainstream, such as nutrition, stress reduction, and lifestyle issues, are now understood to be important and often crucial when combined with scientifically-based, thoroughly researched antiviral treatment. Even if you're not at the point where you need to explore antiviral treatments, you will inevitably be faced with HIV-related health issues and this book contains important information you need to know in order to make critical decisions.

Being HIV-positive poses many unique challenges. The hallmark of HIV infection is its effect on the immune system, but there are other factors involved. As HIV progresses within an infected individual, it also invades many organ systems within that person's body. Since HIV works to destroy a functioning immune system, various unusual infections (known as opportunistic infections) that normally do not cause disease in healthy individuals have a greater propensity to develop. Various other symptoms can easily occur depending on which organ systems are affected as HIV continues to progress. But the good news is that nearly every HIV-impacted individual can be empowered to control the disease and improve his or her health. We now know a lot more about the many facets of controlling HIV, and the quality-of-life has vastly improved for those that are infected. Today you can avoid or overcome the historically pervasive problems once known too well by infected patients during the 1980s and early 1990s. Progress has been made in rapid time: There is little precedence for a disease to have begun with so much tragedy and hopelessness and to have evolved so quickly to what is now being called by many a *chronic manageable disease*.

Huge scientific advances have also been made toward fine-tuning therapy for HIV disease, but it remains a complex, ever-changing dynamic. The number of new drugs to suppress the virus continues to grow as newer classes of agents become part of the treatment landscape. While protease inhibitors and drugs that work by inhibiting HIV from within the cell are considered mainstays of treatment, several newer targets and strategies are being identified. We are now moving toward drugs such as *fusion* and *entry inhibitors* that attack HIV outside the cell. They block the binding of the virus to the CD4 T cell and prevent HIV access to human cellular machinery that is vital to its survival. Other targets such as *integrase,* and new and improved "second generations" of older class agents, continue to make their way and provide further hope for better, more effective treatment. The number of pills needed per drug cocktail and less frequent dosing is also improving with each passing year of research and development. In addition, treatment vaccines and "strategic treatment interruption" are being increasingly investigated.

However, as newer classes of drugs are developed, the potential for long-term problems has grown. A new age of nutritional problems, with a new set of therapeutic dilemmas, has emerged. While wasting was the more prevalent nutritional evil during the early years of the epidemic, today HIV-positive individuals must contend with body shape changes caused by fat redistribution syndromes that occur along with elevated levels of cholesterol and triglycerides. We have also observed an increase in diabetes and cardiovascular complications in HIV patients as they grow older. These are some of the new challenges that physicians and HIV-positive individuals must learn to overcome as we discover more and more about fighting this condition.

As a physician I have always tried to guide patients toward developing a healthy and positive state of mind and to remain steadfast and stubborn regarding health maintenance—this while planning for a long life ahead. Making use of all available tools such as nutrition, physical fitness, reducing stress, and simplifying your life are all keys to successfully managing HIV. I am proud to be part of a book that places a large emphasis on all of these issues, and is in keeping with this philosophy of planning for a long life. *The First Year—HIV* discusses real-life topics like safe sex, adherence to drug cocktails or regimens, proper nutrition and exercise, and the side effects of medications. Brett offers valuable advice to help you avoid contracting other infections or conditions such as hepatitis B or C and herpes that could further complicate your health. He will help you see why counseling and support are important tools in dealing with the psychological stress, depression, and trauma that often accompany an HIV-positive diagnosis and management of the condition in the ensuing months and years. The friendly, easy-to-read language peppered with humor makes *The First Year—HIV* enjoyable reading even as it provides you with important adjunctive strategies that can easily make a huge difference in doing well.

I first became acquainted with Brett during his involvement in starting up the first magazine for HIV-positive individuals and I got to know him during his tenure as editor of *Positively Aware* in Chicago. Brett helped make *Positively Aware* the prominent, nationally respected magazine it is today. It is now one of the finest educational tools available to HIV-positive people, healthcare workers, and physicians. In *The First Year—HIV*, Brett combines his extensive knowledge and insight of HIV disease with a strong passion and vision toward educating and empowering those individuals impacted. This well-written, easily understandable, and comprehensive book is about learning how to handle the issues encountered with HIV infection, and should serve as a reference guide for you and your loved ones. There is more to treatment than medications and antiviral drugs alone. The detailed approach of this book, covering a broad variety of issues, is drawn from many successful patients, experienced physicians, and thought leaders in the field of HIV. This book will inspire you to continue living a long, healthy, and productive life.

DANIEL S. BERGER, M.D., is a Clinical Assistant Professor of Medicine at the University of Illinois at Chicago and is Founder and Medical Director of Chicago's largest private HIV treatment and research center, Northstar Healthcare. He serves on the Board of Directors for Test Positive Aware Network, Chicago's oldest leading AIDS service organization, and is a consultant and regularly featured columnist for its publication, *Positively Aware*. His column, *The Buzz*, is a well-known fixture and routinely featured on TheBody.com. Dr. Berger also serves on the HIV Medical Issues Committee for the Illinois AIDS Drug Assistance Program.

Introduction

I WAS lost when I first moved to Los Angeles. At first, the roads in LA didn't make sense to me. I'm from the Midwest, and highways there usually radiate from a downtown area to the suburbs. In LA, the term is *freeways,* and they connect Sacramento, Palm Springs, and San Diego. When I arrived in LA, I knew that road signs to San Diego meant *south,* Sacramento meant *north,* and Palms Springs meant *west.* That was fine, except there were no signs pointing me to the local Wal-Mart and back.

Soon enough, my friend Nancy gave me a book. Actually, it was a large map, but in the form of a book. It laid out the roads and freeways of LA and I stashed the guide in my car. It helped somewhat. But it wasn't until Nancy began offering her experience and advice that I became at ease with driving in LA. Now, I know to stay off the San Diego Freeway during rush hours. I remember to avoid the freeways near Dodger stadium and the Staples Center before a Dodgers or Lakers game. And I can now find my way to several different Wal-Marts—and get back home.

You might feel lost when you first discover you have HIV. I know when I discovered I was HIV-positive fifteen years ago, I felt lost too. And it was far worse than I felt when I moved to LA. Hearing the HIV-positive news yourself might transform your once-familiar world into a foreign place. You might be wondering: How do I find a doctor? What should I do next? Whom do I tell?

Well, there are no easy answers. HIV is a complicated condition. But there are many common things that people with HIV confront over time. In some ways, this book is a little like a roadmap of those issues. One difference, however, is that it also offers the human element, the experiences, and the wisdom of others who have been in the same boat. Taken together, the two perspectives can help guide you toward more-informed and better decisions today and in the years to come.

What happened to me

I didn't have any noticeable symptoms when I tested positive for HIV at the age of twenty-one. I only took an HIV test because I thought it was the right thing to do. I was shocked when I discovered that it was positive. For many years, the hardest part of having HIV was just knowing that I had it.

For the first few years, my immune system held steady. I didn't need medications. But that eventually changed. Slowly over time, my immune system began to lose the battle it was fighting. As my immune system lost ground, minor symptoms developed, like swollen lymph nodes and skin problems. I felt tired a lot. Over time, I experienced a few more symptoms. I got some irritating warts on my feet; cold sores in the corners of my mouth; inexplicable bruises here and there; and my tongue sometimes burned when I ate spicy foods.

My response to my declining health was to keep closer tabs on the latest medical research. I kept very informed. However, I also knew that surviving wasn't just about gathering information. A *New England Journal of Medicine* article doesn't usually say much about how to talk about HIV with friends and family.

I figured one way to navigate through the emotional and social aspects of having HIV was by talking with other people. Eventually, I met other people who were also HIV-positive, and became close friends with many of them. I learned new ways of thinking about situations I thought were hopeless. Sometimes, I learned valuable details from friendly, informal conversations with other people.

It's not uncommon to live with HIV for fifteen years like I have, and I plan on living to at least age sixty-five—when I can retire. There was a time in the early years of my HIV when I wasn't as optimistic. In fact, I never wore a seat belt in a car back then. "Why bother?" I thought. Now that I'm healthy, I'm far more worried about getting in a car accident on the Los Angeles Freeway than I am about getting sick from HIV.

How to use this book

Unlike a map, this book considers the human element. The chapters are laid out in a way that breaks down the big picture. I have parsed out small, bite-size portions of information that you can absorb right away. The small portions are arranged according to what is most relevant to most people right off the bat. Sometimes I outline the essentials of a complicated topic—like HIV treatment—in an early chapter, and then discuss it later in more detail. The book then moves on to the more subtle aspects of dealing with HIV.

It's great if you got this book on the first day after testing positive for HIV, but it's hardly necessary. If you've had HIV for years, you might be tempted to skip forward. That's fine, but some chapters are like scaffolding around a building. The top part of the scaffolding depends on the foundation at the bottom.

There will be days, perhaps even months, when you'll need a break from thinking about HIV. You might only be able to deal with reading Day 1 through Day 7 right now, and that's fine. You can always come back to the book a month down the road, when your mind has adjusted more. Newly diagnosed or not, I strongly encourage you to start from the beginning and work through the information at your own pace. In some cases, however, your current situation might require you to jump forward to a specific chapter.

Each Day, Week, or Month chapter is divided into a Living and a Learning section. The Living sections focus on the intangible stuff, like emotions, common concerns, or philosophies that doctors use when prescribing HIV medicine. The Learning sections generally focus on a few concrete things you can do—or shouldn't do—to help you stay healthy (such as quitting smoking, improving your diet, or getting more exercise). The choice is always yours, but at least you'll know your options.

Some terms in the book will show up in **boldface**. This means these words are defined in more detail within the glossary located at the back of this book on page 267. You'll also find a few signposts throughout the book. They designate the end of the first seven days, the first month, and first six months. When you reach these milestones, stop and pat yourself on the back, because absorbing this stuff isn't easy.

I will not prescribe

I am not a doctor. I will not prescribe for you. I will not advise you on which treatment I think is best, or how much medication, vitamins, or supplements you should take. That decision is best left to you and your doctor or healthcare provider. Furthermore, HIV treatment changes quickly over time. Every year, new blood tests, drugs, drug combinations, and side effects will continue to emerge. What's right for you today may not be right for you five years from now. I only hope to provide a collection of general principles that have stood the test of time and personal experiences that have helped other people with HIV before you.

Where the focus is

I have focused on things that are relevant to most people who are newly diagnosed with HIV. Of course, if you've had the virus for a longer time, this book is still very useful. It covers a wide range of issues and offers suggestions for anyone affected by HIV.

I have steered clear of many details about HIV medicine. Individual drugs and strategies come and go. For example, doctors at one time thought the best approach was to offer HIV medicine to all people early in HIV disease. This "hit hard, hit early" approach has fallen out of favor today, and has been replaced with a "hit hard, but wait longer" approach. New drugs and new tests may alter things again in the future.

I think it's important for you to know a few things about me and this book. In the past, when I wrote articles for HIV treatment publications, they were often funded by the pharmaceutical companies. Sometimes this fact influenced the information I wrote. I want you to know that this book is entirely funded and produced by my publisher, Marlowe & Company. I myself happen to own a small amount of stock in a pharmaceutical company called Gilead, but I have no other connection with pharmaceutical companies, either financially or otherwise. I think it's important for you to know that. I also think it's important for you to be on the lookout for possible pharmaceutical company involvement in anything you read about HIV.

• • •

Keep on learning

Thanks to a road map and advice from friends, I've learned how to find my way through Los Angeles. In the same way, this book will help you better navigate through the complexities of living with HIV.

People are different and they absorb information in different ways. Some people learn best by listening to or talking with another person. This book will help you locate who can help you, especially with things like healthcare. Other people absorb information through the written word or the Internet. This book offers ways to assess the quality of the information you may encounter.

Some people may slam the door on everything related to HIV. They more or less may choose not to think about the virus at all. Sometimes, a dose of denial is perfectly understandable (certainly, I went through periods of denial). But understand that there are certain times in the HIV disease when denial carries a higher price. If you pay attention to your health now, you might save yourself some headaches in the future. You might have more peace of mind. This book will help you understand what choices and options you may encounter down the road.

HIV Is Manageable

HIV IS a completely different condition than it was a few years ago. Today, things are better. An HIV-positive diagnosis does not mean an inevitable decline in health, as it once did. In fact, the future is bright for people who are newly diagnosed with the virus—and things get better with every passing year.

If you haven't kept up on all the latest progress in HIV and medicine, your positive diagnosis may be quite upsetting. What you've learned about the virus has probably come from news-papers or television. Images of sickly people and hospital beds may be floating around your mind. Those images, however, speak of the old days, before 1996. That's when HIV medicine turned the corner and got dramatically better. And the outlook for people with the virus continues to improve.

You might know a little about HIV or AIDS. Perhaps you even know someone who is HIV-positive. If you're somewhat knowledgeable about the virus, you might be less concerned about your future. Instead, your worries may be focused on other people in your life, people close to you, those who may be less informed than you are. How partners, spouses, family members, or friends will respond to the news may be a bigger cause of worry for you. For now, it's a good idea to focus on you, and take care of yourself.

Testing HIV-positive can be scary. People respond to the news in different ways. Whatever your beliefs about the virus may be, the bottom line is this: Today's outlook for people with HIV is very optimistic. "People with HIV can have a full life and live a normal life expectancy if they do the right things," says Daniel S. Berger, M.D., a physician who has been treating people with HIV for many years.

This book is all about "doing the right things." But what's right for one person can be wrong for another. To make it all more complicated, what's right today may not be right tomorrow. Medicine changes over time. However, the basic rules, general guidelines, and the experiences of many people before you will always hold true over time. This is what you'll find in this book.

Having HIV means many things

Having HIV does not mean you have AIDS. A positive HIV test result means that you have been infected with the virus. Having HIV does not mean that you will feel the effects of the virus immediately, nor does it mean that you have AIDS. Without intervening HIV medicine, the average time between initial infection and the development of the symptoms associated with AIDS is about ten years. However, HIV medicine can add another twenty years or more to the equation.

You might not need HIV medicine for many years. Depending when you were diagnosed with the virus and how your immune system has responded to it, you may not need medicine anytime soon, perhaps not for years. Some people live for fifteen or twenty years without medicine. However, the only way to be sure is to see a doctor and have special blood tests performed. These blood tests can tell you much about the strength of your immune system.

HIV medicine is good now and it's getting better every year. The good news about HIV is not just about the medicine, which, incidentally, is effective and safe when used correctly. The untold story is about all the different blood tests that are available now to help guide your medical decisions. Years ago, doctors made educated guesses about how to fight the virus. Today, new blood tests can describe with precision what kind of HIV is in your body and how well HIV medicine will work for you. Both the drugs and the tests are great reasons for optimism.

You can continue to have an active and full life. Having HIV should not stop you from pursuing the life you wanted before your diagnosis. There are no medical reasons why you can't be just as active as you were before. This includes pursuing athletic goals, traveling to foreign countries, earning a college degree, or achieving success in your job or career. Furthermore, there are no medical reasons why you can't have a traditional family, find a spouse or a partner, or pursue sexual relationships with other people.

You've already taken one of the hardest steps: You had the courage to take an HIV test. This means you've learned the truth about what's happening to you. Now, you're reading this book to learn even more. You are taking control of your health and not letting your health control you.

It's true that things may be tough for you in the next year. The days, weeks, and months ahead may feel like a roller coaster of fears, emotions, and unfamiliar experiences. But understand that you're not alone. Many people have gone through similar experiences. The purpose of this book is to describe the lessons learned from these people before you. These lessons can help you today and in the days to come.

Whatever your initial response was to testing HIV-positive, remember that you have more control than you might think. It's easy to forget. You might choose to jump in and learn everything you can about the virus. You might choose to take a vacation from HIV for a time, knowing you'll deal with things later. Or you might just pretend you never tested HIV-positive in the first. It's always your call. It's up to you to decide what course you want your life—and your HIV—to take.

IN A SENTENCE:

By finding out your HIV status, you're already taking control of your health.

learning

Adjusting to the News

CRYING IS a normal and healthy response after testing positive for HIV. Crying releases tension. In fact, studies show that crying brings down blood pressure, slows your heart rate, and relieves pressure on the cardiovascular system. The message: Let it all out.

"People who actually have access to their deep sadness and who are able to share it with others—these are probably rather healthy people," says Jelka Jonker, a therapist at AIDS Project Los Angeles.

Steve G. is a person who says he generally doesn't cry much. But he describes breaking down in tears after he tested HIV-positive. "I couldn't cry hard enough," he says.

On the other hand, some people feel emotionally numb at first. If you expected a positive test result, the news might bring a mixture of sadness and relief. The relief comes from finally knowing what you've suspected for some time. A positive test might feel like the last piece of a puzzle, and now you can get on with dealing with reality.

Either way, there's a good chance you'll begin to feel nervous, overwhelmed, or even panicky. This feeling is called **anxiety**.

People often deal with anxiety by using alcohol, food, prescription drugs, street drugs, and exercise.

Jelka Jonker says that it's important to feel the emotions, and not simply to block them with alcohol, drugs, or destructive behaviors. She says that you may need to "push through" these emotions as they happen. And there's no specific order as to how emotions will beset you. The emotional roller-coaster ride is quite normal—overwhelming at times, but quite normal.

Feeling nervous is normal

For better or worse, many people often rely on mind-altering substances to cope with stressful events in life. Few experiences are more stressful than discovering you have a potentially life-threatening disease, such as HIV.

For some people, especially those who tend to be nervous or anxious in general, prescriptions drugs known as **sedatives** (Xanax, Ativan, or any benzodiazepine) might provide short-term relief from anxiety. However, if you're prone to substance abuse, sedatives or alcohol might hurt more than help your life in the long run.

There are a few healthier choices for initially coping with the news:

- O **Cry.** Being weepy is for wimps. Try balling with your heart and gut, like what you hear at an Italian funeral.
- O **Comfort foods.** Forget the diet for now. Ice cream, macaroni and cheese, and pizza are generally considered comforting foods. But remember—comfort foods are just a short-term way to cope with difficult situations. A bad diet over time is not good for your health.
- O **Walk, run, hike, or lift weights.** Studies show that regular exercisers adjust better and more quickly to the news of testing HIV-positive.
- O **Creative endeavors.** Try writing or painting. Anything that takes your mind off things for a while—even a good movie—can be a great way to deal with scary feelings.

"The day I tested positive, my best friend brought over two canvasses and some oil paints," says Glenn G. "We sat for several hours and painted. I'm no painter, but I didn't care. Everything in my head was so frenetic, and that's exactly what I painted. It got me through that day, and that painting is still up on my wall today."

IN A SENTENCE:

You'll probably experience some degree of anxiety, but that's completely normal and there are many ways to cope.

Emotional Overload

TESTING POSITIVE for HIV can feel like a slow-motion car wreck for some people. In the hours afterward, you may have felt as though you were watching a movie and the diagnosis was given to someone in the movie. This experience is called **disassociation**. It's a fancy word for how your mind deals with traumatic events. Feeling "separate from yourself" is a normal reaction to very bad news.

For other people, the news is less traumatic. Daniel S. Berger, M.D., medical director at Northstar Medical Clinic, says that people today generally know that effective HIV treatment is available. He says some people might not even take the news seriously, thinking the diagnosis is on par with something like syphilis.

"Maybe they don't realize it in the beginning, but as time goes on, as they learn more about what it means to be infected, it hits them down the road," says Berger. "Sometimes they fall apart and sometimes they don't. At our clinic, we try to have newly diagnosed patients visit with a therapist to be evaluated to catch problems before they get out of hand."

Some people shut down entirely when they first get their HIV diagnosis. A study of people who were newly diagnosed with HIV showed that about one in three delay seeking medical attention for at least one year after their diagnosis. Another one in three people delay seeing a doctor for at least two years or more.

Denial is an option. It's possible to pretend nothing happened. If denial gets you through a particularly tough day, it can be a good thing. But over the course of weeks and months, using denial to cope with HIV will probably make things worse. Research also shows that people who use denial tend to progress faster to AIDS. I'm not saying that denial causes AIDS, but rather that denial can get in the way of your getting proper medical care.

Feel the feelings and talk about them

You will feel many different emotions in the first week after learning your HIV status. "It's usually helpful for people to talk to someone professionally to normalize all those feelings," says Jelka Jonker, a therapist at AIDS Project Los Angeles. She notes that people need to feel the emotions and experience the phases of adjustment.

Many people have gone through the same emotions and fears that you may be feeling right now. Some of the more common fears are:

○ **Fear of the unknown.** You might believe you won't live much longer.
○ **Fear of stigmatization.** You might think HIV will bring labeling, rejection, isolation, or discrimination.
○ **Concern about family.** You may be worried about the well-being of your children, parents, or close friends.
○ **Pressure to maintain a "false front."** You might feel as if you should act happy when you don't feel that way.

You might feel "on your own" with these worries or fears. You're not. Many people with HIV have experienced these thoughts. One way to manage your feelings is by talking with someone who has gone through similar experiences, or someone with professional training, such as an HIV counselor. In Month 3, I discuss in more detail how to find professional help, or at least how to connect with others in the same boat.

Self-blame is another common feeling

Self-blame is also a common feeling at first. You might have known how to avoid HIV but you didn't. This may lead to feelings of guilt or self-hate. "What goes through your mind is 'I should have used a condom' or 'I should have used a clean needle,'" says Mark H. "That whole woulda-shoulda-coulda thinking is completely understandable. The question to ask yourself now is: What am I going to do differently to stay healthy?"

"I'm the kind of person who always says, 'what if' or 'if only.' But I knew that it wouldn't help with HIV," say Rick G. "Try not to fall into this kind of thinking because it doesn't help you, it doesn't accomplish anything. The actions you take and your mental attitude all play a critical role in your health."

It's normal to feel remorse or guilt about some things from the past. After all, remorse and guilt help you make better decisions in the future—and that's a good thing. How many times do you touch a hot stove before you understand that it hurts?

Expect to feel bad at first about getting HIV. But if these feelings of guilt or self-blame eat away at you, or immobilize you for too long, they can get in the way of pursuing a healthier and happier future. Feel the feelings, understand that you can't change the past, and start making better choices in the days to come.

Anger is a normal response

"It's easier to feel anger than to feel shame, guilt, resentment, or sadness," says Mark H. "Sadness hurts, shame hurts, but anger doesn't hurt. You scream and yell and it somehow becomes someone else's problem."

You just found out you have HIV. One day, you're a regular person. The next day, you're different. What about other people who took part in unsafe behaviors? They didn't get the virus. Why did you get it?

Life isn't fair. Different things happen to different people. Sometimes these things make sense and sometimes they don't. If your best friend won a million dollars in the lottery, you might be a little jealous. In a similar way, you might feel angry with people who engaged in the same risky behaviors as you did but who tested negative for HIV. It's completely normal to feel this way.

For some people, this frustration may build up. Without really thinking about it, some people might blame their frustrations on people whom they actually care about. Some people might become angry with people who aren't going through the same thing, such as close friends who have tested HIV-negative.

You may know the person who infected you—or least whom you suspect had a role in it. You may be angry with a spouse or a partner if you believe he or she infected you. It sounds strange, but you might even respond with anger to your spouse or partner if you believe *you* may have infected him or her.

It's normal to think about who infected you, or people whom you may have infected. However, confronting that person is not a great idea during the first week. Unless you're prepared to deal with the consequences of such an exchange now, consider taking some time to adjust to the news for yourself.

In the end, you'll probably find that most of your anger is directed at yourself. If you're the type of person who tends toward self-destructive behavior, you might be compelled to continue engaging in those behaviors. This is to be expected. But eventually you'll get tired of hurting yourself. At some point, the pain of hurting yourself will be greater than the pain of forgiving yourself. When you're ready, there's plenty of help out there.

IN A SENTENCE:

Shock, self-blame, and anger are all common feelings at first.

learning

Be Careful Whom
You Tell

NOW THAT you know beyond a doubt your HIV status, you probably have a desire to talk with someone. Early on, consider keeping the news to a select few until you get a better handle on what's happening for yourself. Telling family members, co-workers, or even some friends might create more problems than it's worth.

The best person to confide in may not be the person who is closest to you. If you have a tight-knit family or social group, or you live in a small community or a rural town, confidentiality is harder to maintain. Consider discussing your diagnosis with people outside of these situations, such as a counselor or trusted friend in another town or city.

Unfortunately, HIV remains a stigma for families and in the workplace. "When it comes to telling your family, it doesn't make a difference whether it was ten years ago or now. Some people have family members with a lot of their own problems," says Daniel S. Berger, M.D., medical director of Northstar Medical Center.

"Also, I think people should not be open about their HIV status in the workplace because other people will be making decisions against them, based on that knowledge. Unfortunately, that's still the reality."

Ultimately, you don't have to tell anyone about your HIV status. This includes family, friends, employers, co-workers, or healthcare providers. Unless there's a compelling reason—say you're a surgeon or a prizefighter—there's no reason why you should tell anyone at work. If you need to leave work early for a doctor's appointment, leave it at that. Otherwise, you risk potentially serious and unnecessary discrimination and disruption.

On the other hand, if telling someone will truly make things easier for you, then the benefits might outweigh the consequences. But before you disclose the news, think about it carefully. Week 3 discusses HIV disclosure in more depth. However, here are a few quick considerations if you are thinking of telling someone about your HIV status:

○ Be clear with yourself about why you want to tell this person. Do you want sympathy, special treatment, or support?
○ Consider the worst-case scenario. Some people may become hysterical. Are you able to deal with that?
○ Give people plenty of time to process the information. Things might seem fine at first, but this can change down the road.
○ Think carefully before telling a spouse or partner right off the bat. It will raise enormous issues for them. (Week 3 gives more detailed discussion on this.)
○ Choose a setting that offers you plenty of time and privacy.

When it comes to HIV, some people prefer to talk to someone anonymously. "People don't just have HIV issues, they often have issues with their sexual orientation, lifestyles, or substance abuse," says Rosetta M., who also works as a health educator in Buffalo, New York. "People need to be hooked up with people who parallel them *and* who have been successful with HIV." Many AIDS organizations around the country offer hotlines, counseling services, and even "HIV buddy" programs. You can find a list of local AIDS organizations in the Resources section at the back of this book.

Unfortunately, research shows that one in five people with HIV regret telling someone. Disclosing the news of an HIV-positive diagnosis is a personal decision and not one to make lightly. During the first week or months, you may be emotionally vulnerable—especially if things don't go as planned when you confide in someone.

There are always unexpected outcomes. "One guy told his friends, and the poor guy lost virtually all of his friends because of it," says Rick G. "It's still an issue, partly because HIV has become so much a part of the landscape that people take it for granted. As long as HIV is off in the distance, it's okay. But when HIV gets too close, when it becomes more than just some figure in a newspaper, that's when people get scared and the bad reactions come out."

Remember that, in most cases, people with HIV have plenty of time to adjust to the news. There's no rush; you're not going anywhere soon. You can postpone telling people for days, months, or even years. When considering whom to tell, take your time. Think about the consequences carefully. Don't tell too many people in the beginning, before you've had a chance to process things for yourself. If possible, you might consider talking with an HIV-positive person first. This way, you can practice what you will say.

Did you know?

○ There are laws designed to protect people with HIV against discrimination in health, employment, housing, and education situations.
○ It is against the law for doctors, nurses, and healthcare providers to tell anyone you are positive without your consent.
○ You do not have to tell your employer that you have HIV.
○ Health professionals are not supposed to treat you differently because of your HIV status.

IN A SENTENCE:

Be thoughtful and selective when disclosing your HIV status—you can never predict how someone will react.

living

A Few Simple Facts

HIV IS nothing more than a virus. The term *HIV* is the abbreviation for *Human Immunodeficiency Virus*. In the 1980s, scientists gave it the "Human" part of its name because only humans can contract HIV. Animals can't get it and you can't get it from animals. However, some viruses are similar to HIV. These unique viruses can infect monkeys and cats. But don't worry; these special viruses can't be transmitted to people. And you can't infect your pet cat with HIV.

Most scientists believe that a long time ago HIV was a very different virus, one that infected only chimpanzees. Because humans ate chimpanzees for food in rural areas of Africa, eventually the virus learned how to survive in humans. In fact, scientists believe the jump from chimp to human happened between 1926 and 1946. The virus probably didn't spread much because people in these rural communities had limited contact with larger cities.

In the 1960s, people from rural African communities began to migrate to larger cities. During this time, the incidence of sexually transmitted diseases, including HIV, accelerated and spread throughout Africa. In fact, old blood samples from a man who lived in the Congo showed that he had died from AIDS-related complications in 1959. HIV found its way to the United States around 1978 as world travel became more common.

HIV is fundamentally different from the virus that once infected chimpanzees. To understand this distinction, imagine your grandparents had several children. Say one of those children moved to another country, got married, and had more children. Now imagine that one of those children knocked on your door. Both of you have the same ancestors, but each of you is from an entirely different family.

HIV is the cause of AIDS

In case you have any doubts, HIV is the cause of AIDS. *AIDS* stands for *Acquired Immune Deficiency Syndrome.* It's acquired because you have to get it somehow. It's not genetic and can't be passed down from generation to generation. The way people transmit HIV is through blood, semen, precum, vaginal fluids, menstrual blood, and breast milk. You cannot get HIV through, saliva, sweat, urine, or feces.

The *Immune Deficiency* part of the name describes how HIV attacks the human immune system. The virus weakens the immune system to the point where other infections and cancers—that ordinarily wouldn't have a chance to make you sick—now have the opportunity to do damage. Doctors call these infections and cancers **opportunistic infections.**

The *Syndrome* part of AIDS describes the fact that AIDS isn't really a disease in a strict medical sense—it is a syndrome, a collection of symptoms. These symptoms are caused by an underlying condition: a weak immune system due to HIV infection. In theory, no one has ever died of AIDS itself. Rather, people die from opportunistic infections that flourish when the immune system is crippled.

HIV is not a punishment

Many people believe that HIV is a "punishment" for bad behavior. This came to light in a study conducted in 2002, which examined how attitudes affect the health of people with HIV. The study looked at things such as depression, quality of life, self-esteem, social support, and coping styles to see what impact they have on the health of people with HIV.

"Attributing one's HIV status as a 'punishment' is a common clinical response from patients," said Steven A. Safren, Ph.D., of the Massachusetts General Hospital department of psychiatry, who led the study. He adds that such "negative beliefs" eventually translate into worse medical outcomes.

Ultimately, the virus is just a tiny piece of genetic material. There are 1,000 to 1,500 different types of virus in the world. Of these, about 250 types cause some disease in humans, including the common cold virus. Now, do you believe that getting a cold is a punishment? Animals get viruses that are similar to HIV. Do you believe that the animals are being punished? Every day, babies are born with HIV. Do you believe that newborns are being punished?

Viruses are found in virtually all forms of life—humans, animals, plants, and even bacteria. HIV just happens to survive best in humans. Once implanted in the human population, the virus just hopped from one person to the next. That's the reality.

Now, how you want to interpret that reality is entirely up to you. Maybe you haven't thought about it. Maybe you're not sure. Maybe it just *seems* like getting HIV is a punishment. And of course, some people in society will insist that HIV *is* a punishment. But it's not. It's just a virus. If you believe those people, at least remember that it's your choice to believe what they say, and it's your choice to continue punishing yourself.

IN A SENTENCE:

Knowing the basic facts about HIV will help you understand that it's only a virus, not a punishment.

learning

Healthy Thinking

PLACE A sick head on a healthy body, and the body will probably follow. Now, place a healthy mind on a sick body. The odds are far better that the body will become healthy. There's power to having a clear, healthy mind—and most people don't tap into or utilize the benefits of healthy thinking.

Every day you make choices. For example, you choose the kind of food you eat for breakfast. You can have a slice of cake with potato chips. On the other hand, you can eat whole-grain cereal with fruit. Now, imagine that you made the same choice every day for ten years. Over time, your choices would add up and have some effect on your health.

In the same way, the choices you make about HIV also add up. It's your choice to see a doctor. Perhaps you've already been to a doctor and you're scheduled to return for a follow-up soon. In both cases, you can choose to avoid seeing the doctor. No one will force you to go against your will. Your immune system may be just fine, so avoiding the doctor may not cause a problem. But if your immune system is weakened, avoiding the doctor has more serious consequences. If you need help finding a doctor, see Week 2 for a more detailed discussion.

• • •

Thinking like a healthy person isn't easy

"Lead the same sort of general healthy life that you would if you wanted to be in the top 10 percent of healthy people." This is the advice to people with HIV offered by Anthony Fauci, M.D., director of the National Institute of Allergy and Infectious Diseases. "You don't want to knock yourself out. You don't want to have poor nutrition. You don't want to *not* do the healthy things in life."

There are commonsense, simple things that everyone should do to stay healthy:

- stop smoking
- exercise regularly
- eat nutritiously
- avoid recreational drugs
- get enough sleep

According to Fauci, there are a few more commonsense things for HIV-positive people to do:

- get a physician or health provider with whom you're comfortable
- never hesitate to get a second opinion
- be compulsive about follow-up care
- lead a generally healthy life
- exercise regularly

"I'm not one to take great care of myself," says Rick G. "But I still try to pay attention to some of the basics: trying to get a good amount of sleep, controlling stress in my life, eating halfway decently. That's one of the most positive and definitive things that you can do. Your actions, your mental attitude about HIV all play a critical role in your health."

Now that you know about some of the basics of staying healthy, does it mean that you will quit smoking and become an exercise fanatic tomorrow? Of course not. Radical changes in behavior are difficult and rarely are they sustained over time. But you can get started, and small things often have big payoffs. Seeing a doctor once every three months is small thing, but the benefit for you as someone with HIV can be huge.

Seeing the dentist on a regular basis is another simple thing that pays off with long-term benefits to your health. Oral healthcare is particularly important for people with HIV. The principles of good oral healthcare are the same for HIV-positive people as they are for those without the virus. HIV is not a reason for you to avoid the dentist.

IN A SENTENCE:

> *Healthy thinking means making healthy choices throughout your life—it will pay off in the end.*

DAY **4**

living

Stigma and Shame

FOR MANY people, HIV is a mark of disgrace. However, the disgrace is in the judgment, not in the disease. The word *stigma* means a "mark of discredit." It comes from an older word, *stigmata*, which is used to describe the wounds of a crucifix. *HIV stigma* refers to the prejudice, discounting, discrediting, and discrimination of people who are perceived to have and do have HIV, as well as anyone associated with them.

In every day life, HIV stigma could mean being excluded from employer health insurance, rejection by friends, mandatory HIV testing without prior consent, or even violence. What's fueling the stigma may be the persistence of inaccurate information. For example, a study found that many Americans still express false beliefs and discomfort about people with HIV and AIDS. The study polled a sample of Americans in 1999, and it found that:

○ 41 percent believed they could get AIDS from using public toilets
○ 50 percent believed that they could get AIDS from being coughed on
○ 50 percent believed they could get AIDS by sharing a drinking glass
○ 33 percent believed that AIDS can be contracted by donating blood

HIV is not transmitted through any of these ways.

On the bright side, the study also noted that the percentage of Americans who actively avoid people with AIDS is shrinking. Support for extremely coercive policies such as mass quarantine of people with the virus has declined dramatically: Only 12 percent in 1999 agreed that people with AIDS should be separated from the rest of society, compared to 34 percent in 1991.

"The belief that AIDS is easily spread and that people with AIDS should be blamed for their illness are important ingredients of stigma," says Gregory M. Herek, a professor of psychology at the University of California at Davis, who conducted the poll of Americans.

"In the early years of the epidemic, most AIDS information programs stressed that AIDS can't be spread through casual contact such as sharing a drinking glass or being around someone who is sneezing," he said. "It's clear that we need to revive those messages and keep reminding people how AIDS is and isn't transmitted."

"Anytime you're around something for the first time, you're frightened," says Rosetta M. She compares the HIV stigma to that of genital herpes. "One in five Americans has genital herpes, but no one knows anyone with herpes. Now, 'one in five' is more popular than Nike—and we all know someone who owns a pair of Nikes."

As with herpes, society views HIV as a "sex" issue, not necessarily a "health" issue. "If I went out and got in a car accident and I got a scar, people can look past it. But if I go out and have sex and something happens, people look differently at that." Rosetta M. contends that many people with HIV have internalized these negative messages, which ultimately leads to feelings of shame.

Shame is bad for your health

Imagine walking into a room full of people who were afraid to touch you. That's how it feels sometimes for people with HIV. You may have a strong defense against the stigma at first, but with time, the negative messages might sink in, and fuel personal feelings of shame.

Shame is a painful emotion caused by guilt, shortcomings, or behaving improperly. According to Jelka Jonker, stigma and shame are especially prevalent among women and the Latino community. "This can happen because [HIV-positive people] are married, bisexual, or gay." Being gay is more difficult within Latino culture, she said. "So there's a lot of stigma there, and HIV is hard to talk about it."

You might feel shame or embarrassment when talking about HIV. This is understandable. But when that shame keeps you from seeking medical care, not letting go of shame will work against you. The challenge, says Rosetta M., is knowing when to cut the shame loose, which she says was probably there even before the HIV diagnosis. She says that for some people, HIV has been a catalyst for confronting feelings of shame. When she tested positive, her motto was: Sink or swim. "I think most of our natures are to swim, even if we only doggie paddle."

IN A SENTENCE:

> *Be prepared to experience stigma or feel shame about your HIV status, which can stem from old, deep-seated feelings that predate your diagnosis or public ignorance about your condition.*

learning

Spirituality
and Religion

THINK OF spirituality and religion as two different circles on a piece of paper. For some people, the circles intersect and overlap. For other people, the two circles couldn't be farther apart. However, what we all have in common is a body, a mind, and a soul.

Obviously, the body is the physical stuff—skin, muscles, bones, and even the genes that were passed along from our parents. The mind is the ability to think, to add numbers, to remember a birthday, and to run from danger, for example, when being chased by a snarling dog.

But the soul, well, that's everything else. It's outside the realm of science and intellect. The soul is the spark of life, the life force, the spirit that makes us want to love, hope for better things, honor truth, or offer compassion. In fact, observing, appreciating, and caring for one's spirit is why many people use the term *spirituality.*

When you initially test positive for HIV, it may feel as if your spirit has been hurt. It's true that your body may be under attack by the virus. Your mind may be in overdrive cranking out scary thoughts. But your spirit is more resistant because it's larger, in a sense, than both your mind and your body.

When you protect your spirit, when you nurture it, or when you show compassion toward yourself, you are being spiritual. It doesn't mean you are being religious or that you believe in God—especially one with a white beard who guards the pearly gates of heaven. For many people, being spiritual can mean being good to yourself in a way that seems to defy reason or the laws of physics.

"I do meditation," says Tim L., who is HIV-positive. He considers himself spiritual but doesn't have an opinion, one way or the other, about God. "I do 'positive reinforcement' of my mental attitude, which is more like a mantra. It depends on the situation."

He positions himself in a relaxed position, maybe against a couch or in a hot bath. "I'll say to myself certain things like 'my mind, body, heart, and soul are in perfect balance,' or 'every day in every way I get better and better,'" he says.

"There's a positive energy in you that needs to be released," says Tim L. "I accept and use my own healing power. I've seen the healing power that people have inside themselves, so I know it's there. I give myself the permission to tap into it, to release it, and to accept it."

Accepting the idea of a healing power within one's self might at first seem foreign or unnatural. But for many people, relying upon such a power within can be a force in coping with HIV.

Faith in God is a healing power for many people

"I believe in God," say Donald W., who is an HIV counselor for the Eastern Regional AIDS Resource Consultation Center in Norfolk, Virginia. He was diagnosed with HIV in 1990, and then diagnosed with chronic hepatitis C several years later. Today, he's a recovering addict, a husband, and a father of two sons. He's also here to send a message to others: If you want to survive, use any means necessary. For Donald W., one of those means is a faith in God.

"Faith has a major role in my life," says Donald W. But it wasn't always that way. Growing up, religion played a superficial role at best. "When I went to church, it was like for Easter—to be dressed up and to been seen."

It was not until many years, after a severe drug addiction and bouts with depression, that Donald W. would begin to build a solid spiritual foundation. "When I went into the rooms of Narcotics Anonymous—which is a spiritual program—we read the twelve steps and the twelve traditions. I kept hearing about a 'power greater than ourselves, a God as we understood him.'" This, for Donald W., would soon become a stepping-stone to the Catholic Church.

So what role does spirituality have in helping people cope with HIV? Perhaps a more objective question is: What are the risks and the benefits of pursuing a path of spirituality?

Faith is a two-way street

In a recent article in the *Journal of the American Medical Association*, Harold G. Koenig, M.D., associate professor of psychiatry and associate professor of medicine at Duke University Medical Center, attempted to shed light on some of these questions.

Pointing to a review of published studies, 66 percent found a "statistically significant relationship between religious involvement and better mental health, greater social support, or less substance abuse."

According to Koenig, many patients have little control over their health conditions, which creates anxiety and, in some cases, furious attempts to regain control. When such attempts fail, anxiety worsens and depression develops. Religious beliefs and practices can provide an indirect form of control that helps to interrupt this vicious cycle. "They enable a patient to turn a health situation over to God and stop worrying and obsessing about it," writes Koenig.

For Precious J., a treatment advocate for Women Alive, an AIDS service organization in Los Angeles, faith has played a critical role in helping her cope with her diagnosis. "It helped me get past the anger," she says, referring specifically to an ex-boyfriend who, she says, infected her with the virus. "With the support of my mom, prayer, going to church, that really helped. I believe—I know—that's why I'm here today, because of my faith in God."

As part of her spiritual evolution, she also points out that faith alone is not enough. "You have to take responsibility for your actions. I just couldn't put all the blame on my ex-boyfriend. I willingly laid down with him without making him put on a condom. That's the part I played in it. I didn't protect myself. I had to get over that part."

Blaming God won't help resolve the problem

Rick G. was twenty-eight years old when he learned his HIV status and doubted he'd reach the age of thirty. "But I had such faith, such good friends, and the love of my family—even though my family didn't know I was HIV-positive. They all kept me going."

According to Rick G., not everyone who had faith before diagnosis maintains it; some people may not be capable of accepting responsibility themselves. "If you can blame God, it takes it out of your hands. This way, you not only get to be the victim, but the angry victim. Sometimes when people feel helpless, they turn to anger to make themselves feel less helpless. The problem is that while you're flailing about in anger, you're still helpless. And those angry people just don't see that."

In the end, everyone eventually wakes up to the same question: How is blame going to help me? How is getting angry with God going to help me out of this? How is blaming myself going to help? Only when you move past blame, Rich G. says, do you begin the process of emotional healing.

Faith is not a substitute for medical care

What's clearly not helpful is when religious beliefs conflict with appropriate medical care. Studies of people with HIV have shown that some stop taking their medications or fail to seek medical care on religious grounds. Religious activities like prayer have been used instead of traditional medical care to treat illness. This poses larger dilemmas for physicians who must monitor patients.

According to Koenig, even if religious beliefs conflict with medical care—as those of Jehovah's Witnesses or Christian Scientists—physicians should be cautious about rejecting them. Instead, he suggests that physicians try to understand the patient's worldview by beginning a dialogue that shows respect for the beliefs and a willingness to work with the patient.

Donald W. concurs, citing a number of philosophical differences that come between his church and his health. "I was fortunate enough to find a church that had an HIV support group. I disagreed with some things that were said there early on and still do. They would say things like, 'Have faith, stop taking your medicine.' I would say, 'Have you lost your mind?'"

As part of Donald W.'s job, he's often asked to speak about AIDS education at schools and churches, which often balk at certain topics. "They say, 'no condoms, don't talk about sex.' They want me only to quote the scripture. Let's get real, people are having sex—all through the Bible belt."

Recent surveys have shown that the southeastern region of the United States is the new "epicenter" of the HIV epidemic. Why? According to Donald W., the reason is primarily the denial about the prevalence of sexual activity and substance abuse "especially in the churches." He said the overriding mantra in the Bible belt is silence, except for abstinence. "That's the philosophy down here: You shouldn't be doing it."

Religion-based denial is compounding the problems

Bob Munk is a seasoned HIV advocate and the driving force behind New Mexico's AIDS InfoNet, an online information Web site. He's concerned that climbing rates of HIV infection in the southeast US are an ominous sign for the region.

The trend, he says, is just part of the stigma that surrounds HIV, especially in the Southeast, where the infrastructure of AIDS service organizations pales in comparison to the region's religion-based infrastructure.

He says religion-based denial "plays into people not wanting to get tested. If they do get tested, they don't want to get treated or to disclose. They don't disclose, so they don't realize that everybody around them has probably got the virus."

It's exactly this sense of isolation that drives Donald W. to continue being outspoken about HIV and substance abuse issues despite the obstacles. It's his faith, he says, that keeps him moving forward. "I wake up every morning. I do my meds. I believe in God. I truly believe in God," says Donald W. "He's walked me through this so far, and he's not finished with me yet."

IN A SENTENCE:

> *Relying upon spiritual tools—whether they are religious in nature or not—can be an effective way of coping with HIV.*

DAY 5

living

Free Services Are Available

YOU MIGHT need some help. You might want some advice about health insurance. Maybe you're having problems with your landlord and you need a lawyer. Perhaps you have a toothache but you can't afford to see a dentist right now. In these cases, the HIV system—sometimes called AIDS organizations—can be a big help.

Equally, the HIV system can seem intimidating at first. These organizations are often highly bureaucratic. Call an AIDS organization and you'll probably get put on hold, transferred a few times, and end up having to leave a voice message.

"The system is enormously frustrating, but cracking the system has saved my life," says Mark H. "Many states have special programs that offer free HIV medicine or affordable health insurance."

AIDS organizations offer special—and often free—services to people with HIV, but to become affiliated with one in your area may require some persistence on your part and plenty of paperwork. If you need professional services sooner rather than later, start the paperwork as soon as possible.

How do you start? Call your state's HIV hotline. A list of state hotlines can be found in the Resources section of this book. Start on a local level. Look to see what organizations are in your neighborhood or in your city. Then talk with people in those organizations to find out more information.

"It all falls back on your own research," says Mark H. "There's not a state in our country where you can't find some resource to help. The Internet is a great source of information. If you don't have access to the Internet, you can always pick up the phone, even if you're in Wyoming."

At least in the larger metropolitan areas, here's the menu:

○ **Referrals for you and significant others**. Say a family member discovers you have HIV and becomes extremely distressed. You may need to find an appropriate counselor for this family member.

○ **Assistance with healthcare or prescription drugs**. Many states offer free or discounted programs to help people without health insurance. A case manager may be able to find various options for you.

○ **Dental care**. Often overlooked, dental care is critical for maintaining the overall health of people with HIV. Unfortunately, dental insurance is not easy to find. Many AIDS organizations provide dental services or offer access to special programs.

○ **Nutrition education and dieticians.** Free or discounted consultations with trained nutrition experts or registered dieticians are provided by many AIDS organizations. Nutrition is especially important if you're thinking about starting on HIV medicine.

○ **Legal assistance.** Say your health insurance company suddenly decides not to pay a $5,000 medical bill. A lawyer may be able to help you force the company to pay the claim or at least negotiate an acceptable repayment plan.

○ **Events and workshops.** Many AIDS organization offer local seminars or presentations on new medicine, emerging side effects, safe sex, dating, or social events.

○ **Mental health services.** Perhaps you received the news of your HIV diagnosis amid other stressful life events. The compounding issues may cause you to be depressed or extremely nervous. Discussing these feelings with a trained therapist can help you work through some of the emotional issues.

○ **Support groups.** Support groups are usually safe places to discuss in detail how to cope with day-to-day worries that come with having HIV.

○ **Substance-abuse counseling.** Not sure if you drink too much? Perhaps you've been experimenting with illicit drugs and you're having trouble quitting. For some people, HIV may be secondary to substance abuse. Drug counseling is available to help with these issues.

○ **Safe, stable, and affordable housing.** If you have children, finding appropriate housing may be a concern for you. Some AIDS organizations offer help in finding low-income housing.

○ **Political representation**. It may not seem important to you now, but it's good to know that people are looking out for the rights of people with HIV as a whole. Money for HIV services and research often comes from Congress, so it's good to know that you are being represented on a political level.

More details about the services offered by AIDS organizations are discussed later in Month 6. If you suddenly find yourself in an emergency, consider jumping ahead for more information.

IN A SENTENCE:

> *Cracking the AIDS organization system can be difficult and frustrating, but it has enormous benefits.*

learning

Frequently Asked Questions

Am I stupid for getting HIV?

It's understandable that some people might feel "stupid" for getting HIV. Society has a way of making people feel bad for some behaviors. But remember, it's not an issue of intelligence, but rather it's a matter of benefits and consequences. HIV is a consequence for a behavior. Along with any behavior comes a consequence. If you engaged in risky behaviors, you'll need to take responsibility for your actions. You may need to let go of the idea that "someone else" has given you HIV. You engaged in a behavior that resulted in your getting HIV. So, you aren't stupid for getting HIV, you just took a risk. The hard part is being responsible for your actions.

What's the difference between HIV and AIDS?

HIV is a virus that infects the immune system and slowly damages it over time. Someone who has tested positive for infection with HIV is referred to as HIV-positive. AIDS is a collection of severe illnesses, which occurs when someone has a much-damaged immune system. Without treatment, many

HIV-positive people do go on to develop AIDS, but this can take ten or so years, depending on the individual.

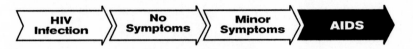

Do possible vaccines change things for people who already have the virus?

No, not really. In 2003, an AIDS vaccine made the headlines as a way to prevent the disease. "The VaxGen trial [one vaccine study that made headlines in 2003] showed absolutely zero efficacy," says Anthony S. Fauci, M.D., director of the National Institute of Allergy and Infectious Diseases. "There was a suggestion in the subset of the analysis that [some groups] might be more protected, but when you do the typical appropriate analysis, that seems to fall through completely. The bottom line is that the trial was not effective at all. Now, that's a first generation vaccine. There are much more complex and likely more successful vaccines in the pipeline, but there really is no guarantee that we're going to get a vaccine for HIV in the near future. I think we need to realize that."

What are the symptoms of HIV?

Without medical intervention, HIV progresses along a predictable course. Within one to three weeks after infection with the virus, most people experience flu-like symptoms, such as fever, sore throat, headache, skin rash, swollen lymph nodes, and a vague feeling of discomfort. These symptoms can last one to four weeks. This initial phase is known as **acute infection**. During this time, HIV reproduces rapidly in the blood and circulates throughout the body. The immune system kicks in and reduces the virus at first, but it can't eliminate it. After acute infection, people usually experience a several-year period without any symptoms at all.

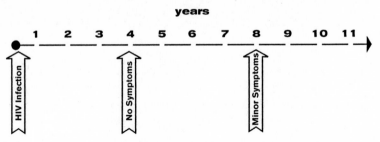

How will an HIV diagnosis change my sex life?

After testing positive for HIV, the vast majority of men and women eventually continue to be sexually active. However, in the first week or month, it's normal to avoid sex. Some even consider celibacy, saying they will "never have sex again." In the first few months after testing HIV-positive, sex may seem awkward for you or your partner. You might feel "dirty" or unattractive to other people, and these feelings may come and go. Eventually, most people learn to enjoy safe sex and adjust to the news. But it's also important to understand that you now have a responsibility not to put other people at risk. It is your responsibility to ensure that your sex or drug partners do not get HIV. It is possible to kill someone by having unsafe sex or sharing needles and you need to know that.

Does alternative therapy help with HIV?

No, alternative therapies do not specifically fight HIV. Many studies have attempted to prove that alternative medicine improves HIV. By all accounts, they have failed to show a positive connection. Some alternative therapies are dangerous and can make HIV worse. However, if you're looking for ways to reduce stress, anxiety, or depression, chances are much better you'll find some alternative therapies beneficial. Some forms of alternative therapy that may improve stress and anxiety include yoga, massage, meditation, and acupuncture.

Why should I trust doctors or pharmaceutical companies?

This requires a two-part answer: First, by trusting doctors, you get the benefit of receiving healthcare, which can help you live longer and healthier. The second part of the answer is: You probably should not trust most pharmaceutical companies. This doesn't mean these companies are bad, it only means that they are motivated by profit, not by social causes. It's always helpful to understand this agenda when reading brochures and pamphlets produced by pharmaceutical companies.

IN A SENTENCE:

Many people have the same questions when they first discover they have HIV.

DAY **6**

living

Consider a Support Group

"I'VE NEVER really been much of the support group type," says Rick G. "Instead, a bunch of us HIV-positive guys get together on Thursday evenings at a bar in Chicago called Berlin. We usually meet after work, have a couple of drinks, and talk.

"In fact, one evening we talked about support groups," says Rick G. "We decided meeting here was the closest thing we have to a support group. Basically, we all have plenty of friends, we have family, and people that we can talk with."

In the first few days, weeks, and months after testing HIV-positive, talking about HIV might not be easy for you. You might not be ready to discuss the issue with your family or certain friends. On the other hand, you might feel isolated and alone.

If you don't know anyone with HIV, one option is attending a short-term support group. Many local health or AIDS organizations offer support groups. Many of these groups are tailored to different needs—such as spiritual guidance and recovery issues—and different populations—such as gay men, women, people of African descent, people of Latino descent, young adults, and family members. Some groups even offer an "HIV buddy" program where newly diagnosed individuals can talk with HIV-positive people of similar backgrounds.

On a more scientific level, here's what some studies say about support groups:

○ Support groups were superior to standard psychotherapy among HIV-positive men with depressed moods.

○ 86 percent of support group participants (men and women) showed significant improvements in "distress severity."

○ Support groups may help people living with HIV maintain safer sexual practices and guide individuals in making positive behavioral changes.

"Don't just go to any support group," warns Rick G. "Shop around. Find out about the organizations that offer these groups. If a support group is sponsored by a hospital, maybe that's too cold and clinical for you. If the group is organized by a nonprofit organization, you might think it's too touchy-feely for you. If you don't like the people in the group, don't go. Find another way."

How do you find an AIDS service organization? It's easier than you might think.

How to find an AIDS service organization

On page 275, you'll find a resource guide of AIDS service organizations. These organizations provide services to people with HIV, and likely offer support groups near you.

The AIDS organizations are listed by state or region. Find an organization close to you. If there are many to choose from, consider the organization's specific location and the kind of people it serves.

If the organization offers a support group, sign up for it, even if you aren't sure you will attend. These groups fill up quickly and might not be offered later. When it comes time for the group, you can always cancel at that time.

If the organization you call does not offer support groups, ask for a referral to one that does. If the organization doesn't know or doesn't return your call, be persistent. Many organizations are more disorganized than you might think.

IN A SENTENCE:

Talking with other people in similar situations can help you come to terms with your own situation.

learning

Needles

LET'S FACE it, some people use needles to administer legal and illegal drugs or hormones. If those people have HIV, it's possible that HIV and other viruses can linger in blood droplets inside the used needles. If these needles are shared, it's possible to infect another person. Many states ban the sale of needles without a prescription. Unable to legally access clean needles, some people reuse them or get used ones from unreliable sources.

Needle-exchange programs are simply programs where clean needles are exchanged for dirty ones. The purpose of this is to prevent the sharing of needles or injection equipment, which prevents HIV and other diseases. Many programs also offer services to participants of needle exchange, including referrals to drug treatment and counseling.

Few needle-exchange programs exist in the United States because many state laws prohibit the possession, distribution, or sale of clean syringes. Most of these laws were designed to reduce illicit drug use. But more than one hundred needle-exchange programs exist in forty communities in twenty-eight states, resulting from a variety of legal loopholes, including exceptions to state laws and special health waivers.

Some people claim that needle-exchange programs worsen the damage caused by injection drug use, or that such programs send the message that "it's okay" to use illicit drugs. On the other hand, some people claim that needle-exchange programs do not increase drug use. The question is: Does the availability of silverware alone cause a person to eat? Would the absence of silverware alone cause a person to stop eating?

In all likelihood, the debate between these two camps will continue. While politicians and activists bicker over the ethics of needle exchange, the message for you is clear: Don't share needles or otehr IV drug paraphernalia with anyone. Not sharing needles will also protect you from hepatitis B, hepatitis C, and other serious assaults to your immune system.

Finding a needle-exchange program isn't easy

Don't expect to find needle-exchange programs in the Yellow Pages. One good way to find a needle-exchange program near you is to call a free, twenty-four-hour-a-day hotline operated by the Centers for Disease Control (CDC):

CDC HIV hotline
(800) 342-2437

The call is anonymous, meaning that you don't have to give your real name. However, be prepared to give the operator your zip code so he or she can try to locate an organization near you that offers a needle-exchange program.

Another option is to call an AIDS organization in your area. A list of organizations is available in the Resource section of this book. If you call, you might start by asking for basic information about HIV. Then, if you feel comfortable, ask about needle exchange programs in your area.

If you can't get new needles, clean them yourself

If you can't get new works, the next best thing you can do is clean them. Here's how to clean your needles and other paraphernalia:

STEP I:

Draw clean water all the way up into your set, shake it, and squirt it out. Repeat that process three times.

Draw In

Shake Several
Times

Push Out

Step 2:

Then do it twice with full-strength household bleach (not diluted). Try to leave the bleach in for two minutes each time.

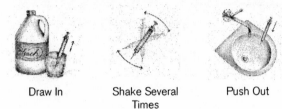

Draw In   Shake Several   Push Out
                    Times

Step 3:

Finally, flush again, three times, with clean water. Clean the cooker by rinsing well with bleach, and never reuse cotton.

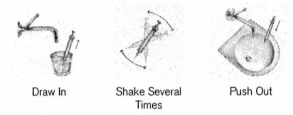

Draw In   Shake Several   Push Out
                    Times

IN A SENTENCE:

If you use needles for any reason, don't share them—get clean ones if possible, or clean them yourself.

living

Tracking Your Health

AT FIRST, you might roll your eyes at the idea of keeping a health journal. Keeping a written log of your health, moods, and medications might seem a little corny, too earthy-crunchy, or "woo-woo" as some on the East coast like to say about those on the West coast. Woo-woo or not, keeping a meticulous health journal is actually a commonsense good idea.

HIV is a complicated disease that slowly affects the immune system over a period of years. At the same time, healthcare in general has become increasingly complex. Your doctor or healthcare provider may not remember every detail of your situation. Furthermore, your primary care physician might refer you to a specialist, such as a skin doctor or an ear, nose, and throat specialist. Keeping a health journal can help you keep track of important blood results that might be handy for specialists.

More than just being handy, a health journal may be what you need to keep from becoming a hypochondriac. Having HIV can make anyone wonder about a simple sniffle or itch. However, **hypochondria** is preoccupation with physical health to the point of obsession. This preoccupation with symptoms is unpleasant and can interfere with daily life in a negative way.

Keeping a health journal can be as complicated or as simple as you want to make it. If you're the kind of person who doesn't like to remember details, then a health journal is even more important. Say, for example, you have a doctor's appointment in two months. Before the visit, you might experience a minor symptom, such as swollen lymph nodes or mild fevers. If you write down your specific symptoms and the dates they occurred, then on your next visit to the doctor you can communicate the symptoms in detail to your doctor with accuracy.

A health journal should reflect the priorities that are important for you. You might want to track how often you exercise or how nutritiously you have been eating. You might be concerned about overindulging in, say, alcohol. You can write down the amount you drink over the course of weeks and months. Reading over your entries at a later time might give you a new perspective on things. Obviously, there's no limit on the details you can track with a journal, but here are a few areas you should consider tracking:

- nutrition/exercise
- key blood tests and results
- previous vaccinations and when they occurred
- your moods or negative thinking
- medications that you take and side effects
- longer-term side effects that can be caused by HIV medicine
- priorities or goals

Nutrition/exercise

Say, for example, you experience recurrent bouts of diarrhea. In this case, you might consider keeping detailed records of all the foods you eat and how they affect you. You might start by recording the time of each meal, what you eat, and how you feel afterward. Make sure that you note every significant symptom or response as it occurs.

Perhaps you decide to embark on an exercise program with a goal of a 45-minute workout three times a week. Over the course of weeks, by tracking your progress in a health journal, you can see your progress over time. You might want to keep track of weights lifted, minutes of cardio, or even exercises that you like versus ones that you dislike. Many people keep food diaries to help control their weight.

Key blood tests

As you'll learn in later chapters, there are some important blood tests for people with HIV to keep track of over time. These results will help you and your doctor assess the strength of your immune system. If, down the road, you change doctors or visit a specialist who might not have your medical records on hand, your health journal can help you maximize your interaction with the specialist. Later on you will learn more about the meaning of specific blood tests, but for now a few critical ones are:

- ○ **CD4+ T-cell counts**: More commonly called T-cells.
- ○ **HIV viral load**: Measures the amount of the virus in your blood.
- ○ **Weight/body mass index**: Can help you see whether you're gaining or losing weight over time.
- ○ **Cholesterol/triglycerides**: These tests measure the amount of special fatty substances floating around in your blood.
- ○ **Liver tests (AST):** These tests measure the health of your liver, and for people who have underlying liver conditions, tracking the health of your liver can help them spot a problem before it gets out of hand.
- ○ **Herpes outbreaks:** If you get cold sores or suspect you may have a form of the herpes virus, it's wise to record where on your body outbreaks occur and how often.

Vaccination schedules

It's not unusual for people to get the vaccines they need from various healthcare providers over the course of their lifetimes. For example, you might have gotten one vaccine from your doctor, and then be vaccinated for something else at a community clinic or hospital. Or, you may change healthcare providers as a result of moving from one region to another. You may not have a central record of your vaccines. This can create problems. For example, two important vaccines for people with HIV are the hepatitis A and hepatitis B vaccines. To make things more complicated, sometimes vaccines must be administered multiple times over the course of months. Keeping vaccination details in a health journal can help take the guesswork out of the process.

Moods shifts and negative thinking

Your moods can change over time. Testing positive for HIV might be something that triggers depression or anxiety in the months that follow. Tracking your general moods over time can be a great tool for monitoring the "health of your head." Sometimes, people who get depressed are not aware of their shifting moods. One day you might feel fine, then suddenly you're feeling sad, anxious, or angry, without knowing why. Mood changes like these may be caused by an "unfelt feeling," which might be traced to an external event. Writing down your moods and perhaps some external events can help you become more aware of your feelings and the things that upset you.

Medications and side effects

Even if you're not taking HIV medications right now, tracking what drugs you do take—and the side effects they cause—might help you sometime in the future. For example, if your doctor prescribed you an antidepressant, you can write down any side effects the drug is causing you. At your next doctor's visit, you can bring the journal and describe in detail the side effects. This way, your doctor or healthcare provider might be less likely to dismiss the symptoms as "in your head" and not worth worrying about. In fact, this works even for medications such as common antibiotics. From keeping a health journal, I've determined that an antibiotic called amoxicillin makes me queasy. Now, if my doctor asks if I am allergic to any antibiotics, I'm able to say "no, but amoxicillin makes me sick."

Long-term side effects

Some HIV medicines can cause certain side effects that can affect the general distribution of fat in your body. It's especially frustrating because these side effects are very subtle and occur slowly over the course of months and years. It might be a wise idea to start with a baseline measurement of your body. You can measure the circumference of your stomach or legs, for example. Then, write the number in your health journal. Six months later, you can take your measurements again and compare the results to see if HIV medicine is causing you any side effects. You could even take a Polaroid picture of yourself wearing nothing but your underwear, and then compare the shape of your body to the Polaroid picture as time goes on. If nothing else, this will go a long way toward easing any worries you have about these side effects.

Priorities or goals

A health journal might also be a good place to write down what's important for you in a larger sense. Obviously, what's important for one person may not be important for another. You might consider taking a few minutes to think about this question. For example, in my health journal I keep a list of general priorities in my life and I rank the importance of each. I keep the list on my refrigerator and above my desk. Whenever I wonder about a difficult or perplexing situation in life, I refer back to this list to see how consistent it is among my personal priorities. For me, they include:

○ *Health.* For me, health comes first above all else. As my grandmother used to say, when you have your health, you have everything.
○ *Sanity.* This is a generic term I use to remind me about stress levels, doing things that are good for my emotional health, or even keeping substance abuse in check.
○ *Relationships.* Some people say that the quality of one's life can be measured by the quality of one's relationships with other people. This priority helps remind me to keep up with friends and family.
○ *Integrity.* Not everyone feels this way, but I find it's important to try to keep my promises and do things that I believe are right for me.
○ *The Basics.* This term describes the importance of keeping up with the basic things in life, such as paying rent on time, making sure I have car insurance when I drive, and keeping close track of my income.

Setting up a health journal is easy and inexpensive

You don't need to spend much money to create a health journal. For less than five dollars, you can find a notebook or a pad of paper at any grocery store. You might want to use a notebook that also has pockets where you can keep related articles or even miscellaneous tidbits, such as health receipts or laboratory reports. First, decide the details you want to track over time. Then, with each entry, be sure to write down the date so that you have a record of any changes. You also might want to write down any questions that you want to discuss with your doctor. Don't forget to bring the health journal with you when you visit a doctor or healthcare provider. Going through your journal is a good way to pass the time while in the waiting room.

Are you a hypochondriac?

The Whiteley Index is a widely used test to determine hypochondria. As with all tests the result must be interpreted cautiously. A high score is an indication that you could profit from talking this over with your doctor. Below

Bob's Health Journal

THERE ARE many ways to use a journal and everyone is different. Here is one example of a health journal that will help you get started keeping your own journal.

NOVEMBER 19, 2003
VISITED DOCTOR ON NOVEMBER 18

doctor visit	May 2	July 12	September 7	November 18
t-cells	376	358	369	320
viral load	12,000 (bDNA)	15,400 (bDNA)	15,100 (bDNA)	17,500 (bDNA)
liver count (AST)	42	38	?	32
blood pressure	140/70	132/80	?	140/75
cholesterol	204	195	197	?
weight	?	205	204	204
symptoms	none	diarrhea	none	none
mood	depressed	okay	depressed	feel fine
general concerns	wondering when to start HIV treatment	doc says minor drop in t-cells is not a big deal for now	my t-cells are up so I feel good	doc says my rising viral load may be reason to consider HIV treatment soon

NOTE: don't worry if you miss some details in one or two visits. The important thing about a health journal is to track the details over the course of months, so you can better see the big picture and the trends over time.

is a list of questions about your health. For each one, circle the number indicating how much this is true for you.

1 = Not at all
2 = A little bit
3 = Moderately
4 = Quite a bit
5 = A great deal

1: *Do you worry a lot about your health?*
1   2   3   4   5

2: *Do you think there is something seriously wrong with your body?*
1   2   3   4   5

3: *Is it hard for you to forget about yourself and think about all sorts of other things?*
1   2   3   4   5

4: *If you feel ill and someone tells you that you are looking better, do you become annoyed?*
1   2   3   4   5

5: *Do you find that you are often aware of various things happening in your body?*
1   2   3   4   5

6: *Are you bothered by many aches and pains?*
1   2   3   4   5

7: *Are you afraid of illness?*
1   2   3   4   5

8: *Do you worry about your health more than most people?*
1   2   3   4   5

9: *Do you get the feeling that people are not taking your illnesses seriously enough?*
1   2   3   4   5

10: *Is it hard for you to believe the doctor when he/she tells you there is nothing for you to worry about?*
1   2   3   4   5

11: *Do you often worry about the possibility that you have a serious illness?*
    1   2   3   4   5

12: *If a disease is brought to your attention (through the radio, TV, news-
    papers, or someone you know), do you worry about getting it yourself?*
    1   2   3   4   5

13: *Do you find that you are bothered by many different symptoms?*
    1   2   3   4   5

14: *Do you often have the symptoms of a very serious disease?*
    1   2   3   4   5

Now add the number from all the questions above. The higher the score, the more hypochondriacal you are likely to be. There is no set cutoff score, but healthy people without health anxiety generally have a score between 14 and 28. Patients with hypochondria are found to have a score between 32 and 55. These numbers are merely indications to help you find out if you have hypochondria. A high score may also signal symptoms of depression or anxiety disorders.

IN A SENTENCE:

> *When you're newly diagnosed with HIV, keeping a health journal
> can help you see the big picture and may help keep you from
> worrying about minor or normal symptoms.*

learning

Take Your
Time to Adjust

TODAY, THERE are good medications that—taken together in various combinations—can slow or even halt the
virus. This will delay—and in many cases reverse—damage to
your immune system.

Most people don't need to start HIV treatment immediately.
HIV affects individuals differently. It's important for you to find
out the health of your immune system. Doctors use special
blood tests to help determine this. (These tests are discussed
in more detail in Week 4.)

Here's a diagram to help make sense of the decisions you'll
face in the future. The entire process may seem complicated,
but if you break it down into smaller parts, it's much easier to
think about.

**You discover
you have HIV**

**Visit a physician or healthcare provider and
have special blood tests taken**

Begin HIV treatment   **Delay HIV treatment**

Decide a strategy, weigh options,   Have blood tests done every
understand what it means   3 to 4 months to check
to take medicine every day.   for any changes.

The decision to begin or delay HIV treatment is your own. Nobody can force you to start treatment. Even if your immune system is severely damaged, you can take certain medications to prevent specific diseases, which may buy you more time to think about your options.

You have the time to make your own decisions. Don't let yourself be pressured into starting treatment, or a particular kind of treatment. Take things slowly, talk to your doctor or other experienced people. Only rarely does the decision need to be made in a hurry. Usually there's a lot of time to consider all the options.

WHAT DOES a 30 percent chance look like? Imagine that the diagram below is a target in a game of darts. Throw the dart once and your chance of hitting the gray zone is 30 percent. If one hundred people throw the dart, about thirty people will hit the gray zone.

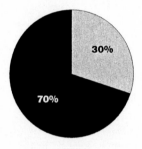

Simply having HIV puts you at a higher risk for getting sick or dying compared to people without the virus. As your immune system becomes more damaged, your risk of getting sick becomes greater. However, you can improve your odds with HIV treatment, which halts the damage to your immune system by stopping the virus. With less virus in your body, your immune system can rebuild itself.

Don't get overwhelmed with the details

You might feel as if there's a lot of information coming at you right now. What's worth knowing? What you need to ask your doctor is (a) how likely is something to happen, and (b) how much does it matter if it does.

For example, coming down with AIDS is bad. However, if your immune system is strong, it's unlikely to happen to you in the next three years. Exactly how long you have depends on how strong your immune system is.

Out of one hundred people with HIV who have strong immune systems, about fifteen will come down with AIDS within the next three years. Among people whose immune systems are damaged, the risk doubles to thirty in one hundred, or 30 percent.

This is a number that you can trust. Researchers have studied thousands of people with HIV. They find a predictable percentage of people get sick over time. Your chances of getting sick relate directly to the strength of your immune system.

IN A SENTENCE:

> *Take your time to make big medical decisions and try not to become overwhelmed by the details.*

FIRST-WEEK MILESTONE

By the end of the first week, you've come a long way in understanding and accepting your HIV diagnosis.

○ YOU KNOW THAT TODAY HIV IS A MANAGEABLE CHRONIC DISEASE, AND, BY TAKING CONTROL OF YOUR HEALTH, YOU CAN EXPECT TO HAVE A FULL LIFE AND LIVE TO A NORMAL LIFE EXPECTANCY.

○ YOU KNOW TO EXPECT A VARIETY OF DIFFICULT EMOTIONS INCLUDING SHOCK, SADNESS, ANXIETY, FEELING "SEPARATE FROM YOURSELF," SELF-BLAME, ANGER, AND DENIAL—ALL OF WHICH ARE NORMAL REACTIONS.

○ YOU RECOGNIZE THAT BEING HEALTHY REQUIRES MAKING HEALTHY CHOICES IN LIFE, WHICH INCLUDES SEEING A DOCTOR ON A REGULAR BASIS.

○ YOU UNDERSTAND THAT HIV STIGMA IS COMMON IN SOCIETY AND MAY LEAD TO PERSONAL FEELINGS OF SHAME.

○ YOU KNOW THAT TALKING TO OTHER PEOPLE WITH HIV CAN HELP YOU BETTER DEAL WITH YOUR OWN SITUATION.

○ You're aware that when you consider taking HIV medicine, you should take your time and understand all the risks involved.

Finding the Best HIV Doctor

IT MAY seem like there's too much information coming your way, people telling you to learn about this, pay attention to that. If you can't deal with too much information, don't. Do something else like watch TV or go see a movie. Be good to yourself.

There's a lot on your mind now. The last thing you probably want to think about is your doctor. The good news is that once you get a good doctor, you can worry a lot less. Maybe you already have a primary physician. Regardless, now is a good time to consider—or reconsider—the person who will guide your HIV care in the future.

Smart patients find smart doctors

Doctors are a little like mechanics. Most people visit a mechanic when something goes wrong with a car. Most people visit a doctor only when they're sick. But the parallel doesn't end there. If you've ever had car troubles, you probably compare your options or shop around, at least a little. Now that you have HIV, it's important that you understand that having a good HIV doctor will help you live longer. Studies have shown this to be true. Think about it: Do you treat yourself as well as you would treat your car?

The number-one advice that Anthony S. Fauci, M.D., director of the National Institute of Allergy and Infectious Diseases, offers people with HIV is to find a trusted physician or healthcare provider. "Get a physician whom you trust, who's knowledgeable and who has experience," says Fauci, "and don't hesitate to get a second opinion."

Patient advocates are pushing these days to make HIV treatment a specific medical specialty with its own training and certification, similar to cancer treatment or diabetes treatment. Advocates say that doctors who don't specialize in HIV are less likely to keep up with fast-changing drug therapies and treatment strategies.

On the other hand, a doctor who focuses only on HIV may overlook the bigger picture. "There are some good points about specific credentialing for HIV because you intensify the knowledge in a particular area," says Fauci. "But I'm afraid if you get too narrow, you're going to wind up keeping out some of the other specialties that you really need to be involved in the total care of an individual with HIV.

"People with HIV need to start thinking not just in terms of HIV—but of the totality of health. You are treating the whole person. You're not just treating a virus anymore. The whole person has lots of other things going on.

"My recommendation for physicians who are going to be—and are—taking care of people with HIV is that it's no longer appropriate to just be an HIV expert," says Fauci. "If you're an HIV expert, you have to be an expert in all the other things that beset a person with HIV."

Find an HIV specialist with diverse training— and whom you like

People have different philosophies when it comes to their doctors. Some people prefer a more aggressive doctor, while others feel more comfortable with a gentler bedside manner. There are trade-offs to each.

The aggressive doctor may be more up-to-date on new HIV research. He or she may even attend HIV conferences or be involved in cutting-edge research studies. HIV treatment changes all the time, so this type of doctor may be able to offer more options. The downside, however, is usually that the aggressive doctor may spend less time with you and your situation.

The warmer and fuzzier HIV doctor may have a better bedside manner. He or she may pay more attention to you, your symptoms, and your worries. This type of doctor may ask about your life in general and how you're feeling overall. In general, this type of physician may be less informed about new medical information or strategies.

Doctors are as different as auto mechanics. If you don't like the guy who changes your oil, you get a new one, right? Finding or changing doctors is obviously not as simple, but that's the idea. Ultimately, the relationship between you and your doctor is a transaction between two people. You get something from your doctor and your doctor gets something from you.

Here's a list of what you should look for when searching for an HIV doctor:

○ **Medical training.** Find a physician who is Board-certified in internal medicine, infectious diseases, or a related specialty. One good suggestion is to phone the potential doctor's receptionist and ask about the doctor's credentials.

○ **Experience working with people with HIV.** Some physicians, particularly in New York and other metropolitan areas, devote most of their practices to treating people with HIV. A doctor who is knowledgeable about HIV will be able to offer you more information and options. Does the doctor belong to the Infectious Disease Society of America or other professional groups involved in AIDS treatment? (If a doctor evades the question, that ought to tell you something.)

○ **Similar philosophies and attitudes.** Some doctors follow a conservative, safe, by-the-book approach to medicine. Others are more willing to try new or alternative therapies. Consider your own philosophies first so you'll know what to look for in a doctor.

○ **Receptiveness to your input.** Will your doctor listen to your suggestions, complaints, or feelings? If you bring information, will he or she read it and respond?

○ **Availability.** Consider the average waiting time for office visits, particularly on your initial visit. Also, think about how quickly your doctor returns phone calls or e-mails. But remember, most doctors are overwhelmed with patients and work. After your first visit, expect to get about fifteen minutes of your doctor's time per visit. (Later in this chapter, you'll learn how to make the most of those fifteen minutes).

○ **Affordability.** Unless you can afford to pay upfront for your medical services, it's likely that your choices will be dictated by the type of healthcare coverage you have. If you have Medicaid, you'll need to find a doctor or clinic that accepts it. If you don't have health insurance, your choices may be even more limited. Call ahead and ask about payment and billing procedures. Work out an acceptable financial arrangement in advance. Remember, you will be monitoring your

HIV for years. Medical bills have a way of stacking up faster than you might think, and in ways you might not expect. Large medical bills can become a problem down the road.

○ **Level of comfort.** You will need to be honest about your lifestyle with your doctor. Your sexual practices and use of recreational drugs will eventually surface as a topic of discussion. If your doctor seems too judgmental, keep searching. It's better to have a doctor who really knows you instead of holding back information.

○ **Follow your intuition.** If you don't like the way a potential doctor runs his practice, continue searching. In the long run, it's better to take some time to find the right doctor than it is to change doctors down the road.

○ **Confidentiality.** Some people are very concerned about keeping their HIV status private. You might choose to get your HIV care from a provider in another town to protect your privacy. You will need to find your own balance between confidentiality and convenience.

A good HIV doctor is hard to find

Not sure exactly how to go about finding a good HIV doctor who's right for you? Below is a plan of action for you. It's one way to organize the process of doctor hunting, which may be obvious to some, but not to others, since most people don't think much about doctors until they're sick. Either way, you will be developing a long-term relationship with your physician. The more advance planning you can do now, the better chance you'll have finding a good HIV doctor. And having a good HIV doctor can translate to living longer and better.

Step 1
Remember that your ultimate goal is to find an HIV-smart doctor with whom you're comfortable and you can afford to see regularly. It might help to make a list of specific traits you want in your doctor.

Step 2
What specific things could prevent you from finding your perfect doctor? One obstacle might be an understandable fear of discussing HIV or sexual issues with unfamiliar people. Another roadblock might be not having health insurance. Now, write down—or at least think about—anything that might block you from getting what you want in Step 1.

STEP 3

Now, pick one obstacle and creatively think about how to get around it. Write down the ways in which you imagine sidestepping all the obstacles you listed in Step 2. For example, if you're uncomfortable discussing sex or recreational drugs with your doctor, one solution might be interviewing several doctors until you come across one who seems "in tune" with those issues. Another example might be a lack of health insurance. There are plenty of ways to get insurance but it takes research and effort on your part. Or you might choose to find a public health clinic that offers HIV care. Either way, try to imagine a way to get what you want—even if you don't have the emotional courage or the money right now. Life has a funny way of changing for the better, if you're receptive.

STEP 4

Call several local AIDS organizations and ask them for physician referrals. There's a list of AIDS organizations on page 275. In most cases, the organization will only give you a list of doctors, their names, numbers, and addresses, nothing else. The organization may not want to favor one doctor over another. Make a list of five or six potential doctors.

STEP 5

If you have any friends with HIV, ask if they are familiar with the doctors on your list. Also, ask them for recommendations and find out how they selected their HIV physician. If you don't know anyone with HIV or don't want to discuss the subject, go online or try calling the doctor's office to see what you can uncover. Remember to ask specifically about insurance and billing procedures. This will help you narrow your list to maybe two or three.

STEP 6

Make an appointment with your top choice, but commit yourself to interviewing at least one other doctor. This way, you'll be able to compare the two. Make clear that you just want to get to know the doctor. Most doctors' offices are—or should be, anyway—receptive to this request. Sometimes these initial consultations are free, but not always. You'll know it when you find the right doctor.

Your doctor is not your friend

Once you've decided on a doctor, schedule an initial visit. Remember, your doctor is not your friend; he's your doctor. There's a lot of talk these days about developing a "doctor-patient relationship." This concept is great in theory, but in reality, the relationship is a transaction. Your doctor is getting paid, either by you, your insurance company, or the government, to keep you healthy.

There's a myth about "special relationships" between doctors and patients. However, competition for shrinking healthcare dollars, the growing numbers of health maintenance organizations (HMOs), and the push toward the "managed care" model of practice have long ago smashed this myth. "Managed care" refers to a variety of techniques for influencing healthcare providers and/or patients. The overall aim of managed care is to contain the cost, the quality, or the access to certain expensive health services.

In fact, some forms of managed care offer a financial incentive for doctors to spend less time with each patient. For instance, some preferred provider organizations (PPOs) may pay less to doctors per patient, but will promise them more patients instead. What this means to you is less time to talk to your doctor.

According to surveys published in the *New England Journal of Medicine*, American physicians spend an average of eighteen to twenty minutes with each patient. My fifteen-year experience of seeing HIV doctors on a regular basis is that, after the initial visit, you're lucky if you get fifteen minutes. But it's not necessarily a bad thing; it's just a reality to which you'll need to adjust.

Making the most of your fifteen minutes requires advanced planning on your part. At some point before your appointment, make a list of topics to discuss. Keep the list in your pocket and carry a pen or pencil with you during the visit. Check off the items on your list as your doctor addresses them. You may feel weird or awkward about this at first, but your doctor will soon learn that you mean business. He or she will likely perceive you as a more organized, directed patient and, therefore, will be more likely to address all of your concerns. Try this just once with your doctor and you'll notice the difference.

Expect to talk a lot during the initial visit

So that you know what to expect from your first official visit, be prepared to discuss:

○ **Your health history.** Your doctor will ask when you first tested positive for HIV and if you have any symptoms, such as fevers, night sweats, weight loss, diarrhea, skin rashes, or changes in your mental status. Be prepared for questions about sexually transmitted diseases, chicken pox or shingles, viral hepatitis, bacterial infections, gynecologic problems, and exposure to tuberculosis (TB), and where you've lived or traveled.

O **Sexual practices**. You will be asked about behaviors that might lead to further transmission of HIV. Your doctor will probably want to know if your sexual partners are aware of your HIV status. You'll probably be encouraged to inform your partners of your HIV status (see Month Two for more discussion on this). You are also likely to get a lesson on condoms and safer sex practices.

O **Recreational substances and/or injecting drugs**. You may be asked about how much alcohol you drink, if you smoke marijuana, or use "party" drugs. If a doctor suspects you inject drugs, you'll probably be asked about your drug-using practices, your source of needles, whether you share needles, and if so, with whom.

O **Depression.** Depression is common in people with HIV. Your doctor may ask about changes in mood, libido, sleeping patterns, appetite, concentration, and memory. Also, your doctor will probably ask whom you have informed of your HIV status and what kinds of support you have. This discussion may include questions about partners, children, family, living situations, and work environments.

Expect a little touching during the physical exam.

During a first visit, you should expect a complete physical examination. Your doctor should look at your skin and inside your mouth, feel your lymph nodes and certain areas near your stomach, and listen to your lungs as you breathe in and out. Your doctor might even want to examine your anus, penis, or vagina.

First visit checklist

A good HIV doctor should perform a number of tests on you. But depending on your situation, you may not have access to a good HIV doctor. Just in case, here's a list of the most important tests you should ask about on your first visit:

O Repeat HIV test. If you were tested anonymously or don't have documentation of your HIV status, your doctor might repeat the HIV test. HIV tests are extremely accurate but false positives can occur from clerical errors.

- ○ HIV viral load. This test measures the amount of the virus in your blood (further chapters discuss this topic in more detail).
- ○ T-Cell (CD4+) counts. This gauges the status of your immune system (further chapters discuss this topic in more detail).
- ○ Complete blood count. This test examines different aspects of your blood.
- ○ Syphilis test. It's possible to have this sexually transmitted disease and not know it.
- ○ TB testing. It's also possible to have been exposed to TB and not know it.
- ○ Toxoplasmosis testing. This is a common infection that people can get through raw meat or handling cat litter.
- ○ Viral hepatitis. You and your doctor will want to know if you have been exposed to hepatitis A, hepatitis B, and/or hepatitis C.
- ○ Gynecological tests. Women with HIV are at increased risk for a number of gynecological problems. Make sure you get a pelvic examination with Pap smear.
- ○ Other lab tests. Depending on your age, sex, and other variables, there may be further tests your doctor will want. Consider a "type-specific serological test" for herpes and an anal Pap smear for men and women.
- ○ Vaccines. There are a number of important vaccines that you can ask about. They include:
- ○ pneumonia
- ○ hepatitis A
- ○ hepatitis B
- ○ dT (tetanus booster)
- ○ influenza vaccine

IN A SENTENCE:

Shop around before choosing an HIV doctor, and make the most of your limited time with that person.

learning

The Virus Versus You

MOST PEOPLE think viruses are creepy. You hear about this virus or that virus and rarely are they good news. So why bother to read more about HIV? If your goal is to live longer and better—and you're facing a medical challenge—you should ask a lot of questions, especially of your doctor.

You'll pose better questions and you'll get better answers if you appear to have a good medical vocabulary. But don't worry too much if you don't understand all the words and phrases associated with HIV right now.

However, if you're anything like me, words like **pathogenesis** make me want to run. When I start reading technical literature, I always manage to find distractions like cleaning my room or chasing flies with the DustBuster.

Here's a brief look at how the Human Immunodeficiency Virus (HIV) works.

HIV is a little like a terrorist

The drama begins when HIV somehow finds its way into the bloodstream, where it floats around for a while undetected. At first, you might think HIV is a smart virus. To the contrary, it's actually dumb compared to other viruses. What HIV has on its side is luck. It's a lucky virus because it always manages to find what it needs to survive.

Meanwhile, back in the bloodstream, the invader eventually sets off an alarm. This alarm, in a simple sense, is the creation of antibodies. Think of antibodies as similar to early-warning sentinels who scour the countryside looking for potential troublemakers. When an antibody sees trouble, it reports it back to immune central. And it always remembers the bad guys.

With the antibody alarm tripped, the immune system is made aware of an illegal break-in. Think of your body as a country or nation. In this analogy, the human immune system is a like a country's department of defense. The immune system defends your body from attack.

This immune defense responds by sending out an army of white blood cells, also known as **T-cells.** Ordinarily, T-cells are excellent soldiers. They're a critical part of the body's first and most robust response to foreign invasion. Different T-cells have different skills, but working together, the army is almost always successful.

One important and unique type of T-cell is called the **CD4 cell**. It makes up the bulk of the body's immune defenses. As fate would have it, HIV prefers to infect CD4 cells—the very cell designed to defeat foreign invaders. In fact, the virus easily enters the CD4 cell and actually uses it as a hideout and a place to grow.

Hiding inside the CD4, HIV then hijacks the cell's DNA factory. The virus uses the cell's own DNA to produce replicas of itself. Imagine if a foreign invader took control of a country's own bullet factory to make more bullets! Not bad for a dumb virus.

With a lot more replicas of itself, HIV bursts out of the T-cell factory, looking for more conquests. Eventually, the T-cell dies. Generally speaking, this process takes about two and a half days.

HIV is fortunate in that it multiples in great numbers. Within twenty-four hours, HIV reproduces itself about ten billion times—roughly equivalent to creating twice the number of all humans on the earth each and every day. Compared with other viruses, HIV's replication rate is high. This gives it a distinct advantage called "resistance," as you'll learn in later chapters.

Size up your enemy by measuring your viral load

The amount of virus swimming in the bloodstream is called the viral level or, more commonly, **viral load**. A high viral load means there's a lot of HIV in the blood. An undetectable viral load is a good thing, because it means there's very little virus in the blood. An undetectable viral load does not mean you can't give the virus to someone else.

In general, the viral load test measures how fast HIV disease is progressing. If someone has a high viral load, HIV is very active, and vice versa. On the other hand, the CD4 cell count reflects how far HIV disease has progressed. In general:

A good thing
High T-cell counts (not very far)
Low or undetectable viral loads (not very fast)
A bad thing
Low T-cell counts (progressed far)
High viral load (progressing fast)

There's a war between your immune system and HIV

There's an ongoing war between HIV and the immune system. During the course of infection, however, this balance of power shifts from side to side. During the first few days of infection, HIV gets the upper hand. This is called acute infection. During an acute infection with HIV, many people report symptoms similar to those with flu.

Once the immune department gets busy, the balance of power is restored. Within months of acute infection, the amount of HIV in the blood is generally reduced and the immune system holds back the virus. This extraordinary balance of power can go on for years.

At some point, however, the immune system begins to run short on soldiers. This leaves HIV with the ability to replicate uncontrollably and to ultimately destroy any remaining T-cells. Without disease-fighting T-cells, the human body is fair game for a host of other unfriendly invaders, ranging from irritating to life-threatening.

By the way, the above process of how HIV does damage is called *pathogenesis*. There, that wasn't so bad. Now for the good part.

Call in your secret weapons when you need help

Antivirals are chemical compounds that, for one reason or another, can interfere with viruses. Specifically HIV is a type of virus called a **retrovirus**. As such, chemical compounds that work against HIV are **antiretrovirals**. I find the word intimidating and hard to read, so I'll just continue using "antiviral" to describe a chemical that slows HIV.

Remember the analogy of the immune system being the department of defense? In this case, antivirals would be like spies. At any point in the conflict between the immune system and HIV, the antiviral spies can be called in. However, the spies don't answer to your immune system, they answer only to you. You decide when the time is right.

Different antivirals are designed to accomplish different tasks. Some antivirals infiltrate the DNA factory and render it useless. Hence the virus can no longer make copies of itself. Other antivirals prevent the final assembly of newly manufactured particles of virus. A more detailed discussion of the antiviral classes will come later. For now, I'll just introduce you to the four major players on the antiviral block:

- ○ nucleosides (or nukes)
- ○ non-nucleosides (or non-nukes)
- ○ protease inhibitors (pronounced *pro-tee-aze*)

None of these drugs is good enough to work alone against HIV. The best way to use these drugs is to combine them in different ways. This is called **combination therapy,** and you've probably heard it referred to as the "**AIDS cocktail**." Another name is **highly active antiretroviral therapy (HAART)**. The term *HAART* first cropped up in HIV lingo because some drug combinations were not considered "highly active." Today, the antivirals and the combinations are vastly improved.

IN A SENTENCE:

> Armed with a good HIV specialist and a basic understanding of how HIV operates, you're on the road to making better choices for a healthier and happier life.

Dealing with People: Disclosing the News

IT'S EASY to imagine a time when HIV test results will be delivered over the Internet: "You've Got HIV." Today, some people get their results by US mail or telephone. No matter how you received your HIV diagnosis, eventually you'll find yourself having a conversation about HIV with someone else.

The thought of disclosing your HIV status to certain people in your life may make you nervous. The good news is that you don't have to tell everyone. You can be selective about whom you tell. It's only been a couple of week since you've been coming to terms with the news yourself. Cut yourself some slack for now.

When you're ready, you'll want to think about deciding whom to tell and whom not to tell. Of course, there's no rule about this because it will change for you over time. This week, you might tell a trusted friend. Next month, you might tell strangers in a support group. Down the down the road, you may tell your parents or your children. Or you might choose never to tell anyone.

The decision to disclose your HIV status to others is always and only yours. However, everyone has their opinion on the subject. Some groups claim the only deciding factor in telling other people is whether or not other people come in direct contact with your bodily fluids such as blood, semen, or vaginal secretions. Others say it's good to tell friends or family for support.

Whatever people say, the reality is that people with HIV are selective about disclosing their health status. According to one study, the process of choosing which individuals to tell the news often involves anguish and uncertainty. Another study found that HIV-positive people were often indecisive about disclosing their HIV status.

How we feel about disclosing our HIV status

- ○ 40 percent report indecision about HIV disclosure
- ○ 31 percent planned never to tell certain people
- ○ 28 percent desired to reveal their status to someone
- ○ 21 percent regretted having told someone

Why disclose your HIV status?

The reasons to disclose one's HIV status will be different for everyone. Whatever your specific reason for wanting to tell someone, chances are good it will fall in one of several general categories. They include:

- ○ the "right" for others to know
- ○ need for emotional support from others
- ○ access to medical resources or services
- ○ the need for intimacy
- ○ integrity

There are pros and cons to disclosing your HIV status

Who should you tell the news that you're HIV-positive? The answer to this question depends on what you want from the person whom you're thinking about telling. You might tell a spouse or partner for emotional support or for his or her own health. You might decide not to tell your children because they're not old enough to grasp "adult" ideas.

Think carefully about whom you tell. As it turns out, about one in five people regret telling their HIV status to someone. The following are some risks and benefits to disclosing your HIV status:

Spouse/partner

Potential benefits: If you have a husband, wife, boyfriend, girlfriend, long-term partner, or whatever you call it, you may find comfort in the support that person can offer. Perhaps your other half can do some of the chores around the house. Maybe they can listen to your worries and give suggestions. Maybe they can pick you up from the doctor's visit. Maybe they'll just listen to your feelings.

Potential Risks: It's possible that your partner may become alarmed by his or her own HIV status. Instead of being supportive, your primary partner may feel nervous about himself or herself. If the two of you aren't getting along these days, an HIV-positive diagnosis in one or both of you is likely to further strain the relationship. Of course, this isn't a suggestion to avoid a rocky relationship by keeping secrets, but if your love life is already on the rocks, consider the timing of telling your partner. You need to cope with the news first. A little "time away" for you to get your own head together might be appropriate.

FRIENDS

Potential Benefits: Studies show that most people disclose their HIV diagnosis to close friends or current partners within days of first learning the news themselves. A close friend may be able to offer new ways of thinking about your situation. He or she may be the best form of support for you by simply listening to you.

Potential Risks: Some people are more informed about HIV than others. A friend may appear comfortable with the news at first, but may turn out to be uncomfortable with that news in the long run. There's no shortage of stories about "friends" disappearing after learning of one's HIV status.

DOCTORS AND DENTISTS

Potential Benefits: Disclosing your HIV status to an HIV doctor should be easy enough. However, people often encounter different types of doctors. While there's reason to tell your primary care physician, there's no reason why your foot doctor needs to know. Dentists are a different story. In theory, your dentist should be using what's called "universal precautions," which are special procedures to avoid any kind of virus, not just HIV. While you're not legally bound to disclosure to your dentist, he or she may be able to help identify certain health problems.

Potential Risks: As with counselors, some doctors may be required by law to report certain events. The regulations vary among states, cities, hospitals, HMOs, and individual practices. By telling a doctor, you risk losing a degree of privacy. As for some nurses and other healthcare workers, like it or not they might be uncomfortable working with someone who they think has HIV.

THERAPISTS AND PSYCHOLOGISTS

Potential Benefits: The benefits of talking to a therapist, social worker, psychologist, or psychiatrist about HIV can be immense. You will probably find comfort in having an objective person to talk with about any number of personal issues that you may be confronting. Some of these issues may include substance abuse, sexual identity, pregnancy, and relationships. My experience has been generally good in terms of disclosing my HIV status to therapists and psychologists. In fact, an experienced social worker or therapist is very likely to offer the best support for you right now.

Potential Risks: If a social worker, therapist, or "shrink" lacks experience with HIV and related issues, you might find the opposite of comfort. It's possible he or she might guide you in a direction that is not productive for you now. You may not be emotionally ready to deal with certain topics. You may disagree about sexuality, religion, spirituality, or morality. These disagreements may cause unnecessary conflict for you at the moment and you'll end up avoiding therapy altogether. If you find yourself too uncomfortable, or even offended for some reason, speak up and terminate the relationship.

SEX PARTNERS AND ONE-NIGHT STANDS

Potential Benefits: The case for disclosing your HIV status to a potential sex partner or one-night stand has little to do with the other person. It's about you and how you conduct yourself in life. Of course, conventional wisdom holds that people with HIV are supposed to inform other people before having sex with them. Besides social and peer pressure to disclose, some state laws actually make it a crime not to disclose.

But laws that attempt to control sexual behavior usually have other motives than protection of public health. If you're having safe sex with other people, the risk to them is low, so there's no moral imperative to uphold (see Month 2 on risks of sex). Besides, what matters morally—ultimately—is what you do sexually, not what you say. The real benefit of disclosing to sex partners comes from having the strength of character to be honest in difficult circumstances. Going through life being ashamed about certain aspects of your life has a funny way of making those aspects of your life truly shameful.

Potential Risks: Telling people you have HIV before having sex with them almost always changes the way people behave sexually. You're more than likely to encounter some negative response, if not outright rejection. They may become afraid to have sex or even to kiss. Although a lot of people these days know about safe sex and how the virus is transmitted, there's still a great deal of stigma and fear. Even if you try to educate people about the topic, their emotions may be too strong. Irrational fear is a hard thing to overcome. If you're a person who gets hurt easily by rejection, you have a tough road ahead of you.

PARENTS

Potential Benefits: If your parents are living and you have a good relationship with one or both of them, your disclosure about being HIV-positive may lead to a stronger relationship in general. Think about it, if you had a child who tested HIV-positive, would you want to know?

Potential Risks: Sometimes parents can have so much emotional investment in your well-being, the news may devastate one or both of them. You may find yourself having to educate them about HIV or provide them with emotional support—and if you're not ready for this, it may add more stress. If the relationship with your parents is less than perfect, the news will most likely worsen the relationship.

SIBLINGS AND CLOSE FAMILY MEMBERS

Potential Benefits: Statistically, family members are usually the last to be told about someone's HIV status—unless that family member is also a friend. You may have a brother, sister, uncle, aunt, or extended family member with whom you can share the news. Disclosing your HIV status may help you feel less alone. Some HIV-positive people tell their brothers and sisters before telling their parents.

Potential Risks: A close family member may be less educated about HIV and the ways people contract it. For example, a sister may take the news in stride until she has her first child. At which point, she may think twice about letting you play with the baby. In addition, although some confidantes may feel privileged and will offer support, others may feel burdened, such as the sibling who must now conceal your HIV status from your parents.

CO-WORKERS

Potential Benefits: You may have friends with whom you work. (I'll discuss employers later.) They might provide an opportunity for you to discuss your health concerns as they relate to your work.

Potential Risks: People love to gossip, especially about co-workers. Like it or not, it happens. You may tell a co-worker about your diagnosis in confidence, only to later find that confidence broken. Work settings are basically rumor mills. Tell the wrong person and you might as well make an announcement at the company picnic.

One Man's Experience:

"Mom, Dad . . . the good news is that I'm gay."

AT AN HIV support group, I met this guy named Eric. He was having a hard time telling his parents that he was HIV-positive. The primary obstacle, as he explained it, was that his parents didn't know he was gay. At the time, Eric was about twenty-four years old and had been having sexual encounters with other men for about three years. At the support group, he rehearsed what he thought the conversation might be.

He had called them in advance and told them there was something important he wanted to tell them. He had planned to spend only one afternoon at his parents' house and break the news during that time. A week later, he reported back. He had gathered his parents around the kitchen table and, after some small talk, he broke the news: "Mom, dad, the good news is that I'm gay." Before they could respond, he then declared that he was also HIV-positive. His mother broke down in tears. His father was stone cold. Eric gave his parents some articles and brochures about HIV and then left.

In the weeks that followed, the relationship between Eric and his parents was stormy. After several months, he reported that his parents eventually adjusted to the news.

IN A SENTENCE:

It's always your own choice to tell other people about your HIV status, so be selective and think carefully about the risks and benefits of disclosing.

learning

Urban Legends, Myths, and Anti-AIDS Propaganda

A guy's friends throw him a twenty-first-birthday party. They get him drunk and chip in for a hotel room and a prostitute for his present. In the morning when this guy wakes up the prostitute is gone. When he goes to the bathroom, written on the mirror is "Welcome to the World of AIDS."

THIS IS not a true story. It's an urban legend. No evidence exists that anything similar to this horrifying tale truly took place. Nonetheless, it was anonymously posted on the Internet in 1994 and proliferated much like a computer virus. Since then, HIV and AIDS have been the subject of countless urban legends over the last twenty years. One favorite of mine is:

Drug users are now taking their used needles and putting them into the coin return slots in public telephones. People are putting their fingers in to recover coins or just to check if anyone left change. They are getting stuck by these needles and infected with hepatitis, HIV, and other diseases.

For some reason, I now think twice before recovering my change from the phones at the airport. Politically correct or not, legends and myths persist because they appeal to human nature. The value of these so-called lessons is not in the storylines; it's in the people that read them. Legends and myths about HIV just reflect the ways that our society feels about HIV.

Fiction appeals to human nature

The tawdry or the terrifying has forever appealed to human nature. So, if you come across something about HIV, consider what you think is a fact and, conversely, what you think is someone's opinion. Most importantly, consider the source. What is the motive of that source supplying the information?

You'll encounter different kinds of information about HIV. Your doctor may offer you advice. Maybe you will come across an informational Web site on the Internet. Perhaps you will read an article or see an advertisement in a local or community newspaper. Some of that information will be good and some bad. Some information will apply directly to you, while much of it won't.

Keep in mind that it's a free country. We like freedom of speech here in the United States. Compared to citizens in other countries, we are afforded a good deal of freedom, especially for the press. Like it or not, most everybody is allowed an opinion. Conflict happens when people express their opinions disguised as fact. Any bozo with thirty-five dollars can create a Web site to promote an opinion or advertise a product. But that doesn't mean you should believe his or her claims.

Here's a checklist for assessing other people's advice, opinions, or information:

○ What part of the message is true? What part actually exists?
○ What part of the message is someone's opinion?
○ What's the motive of the source?

AIDS conspiracies persist because they're good fiction

Conventional wisdom about HIV in the United States holds that HIV causes AIDS. Most people agree this is true. It does so by depleting the immune system, which leaves the human body vulnerable to opportunistic infections. But this wasn't always conventional wisdom.

There was a time when researchers didn't know that HIV was responsible for AIDS. In the early 1980s, researchers suspected that a newly discovered virus had some association with a growing number of sick people, but the suspicions were not proved scientifically until much later.

These days, there's indisputable research to say that HIV causes AIDS. Think about it: Since the introduction of HIV viral load testing and reliable antiviral drugs, the death rate from AIDS has dropped dramatically.

The 1980s and the early 1990s—before new techniques and good HIV drugs—were a grim time for people with HIV and AIDS. Out of despair, many people sought alternative viewpoints. In 1987, Professor Peter Duesberg, of the University of California, Berkeley, vocalized his suspicion that HIV was not the cause of AIDS, basically saying there wasn't sufficient evidence to make the claim.

With passing years, studies have repeatedly disproved Duesberg's claims. Today, the mainstream medical community considers him to be a crackpot at best, and a danger at worst. Nonetheless, his followers adopted Duesberg's theory. Over the years, fringe groups have grown, feeding on suspicion.

Today, the suspicion that HIV does not cause AIDS is alive and well—and more commonly referred to as the "AIDS myth." The AIDS myth is the theory that HIV is actually a harmless virus, doing nothing more than piggybacking on your body.

"Toxins" do not cause AIDS

If the AIDS myth is true, then you're stuck with the problem: What causes AIDS? Duesberg proposed a "toxicological explanation" for the epidemic. "Toxicological" was Duesberg's way of saying "poison." Over the years, Duesberg's "poison-causes-AIDS" theory has taken several turns. In 1997—before success with the AIDS cocktail was documented—Duesberg

---

Word Games: Pick Your Poison

TOX OR TOXI — prefixes that relates to the word poison

TOXIC — describes a substance that is poisonous

TOXICITY — state of being poisonous

TOXIN — a poisonous substance made by your own body

TOXICOLOGICAL — anything related to poison

TOXICOLOGY — a science that deals with effects and problems of poison

---

wrote about what he called the "drug-AIDS hypothesis." In it Duesberg claims that the use of recreational drugs, like cocaine, crystal, poppers, and heroin, is a cause of AIDS. Another source of AIDS, he says, is the same antiviral drugs designed to stop AIDS. The height of Duesberg's popularity was just before new HIV treatments dramatically improved treatment. And over time, Duesberg's outdated "which came first, chicken or egg?" hypothesis has been disproved again and again.

Beware of "Anti-AIDS" cults

You just got hit with an HIV diagnosis so you're probably seeking answers or comfort. You may be more susceptible to ideas that, under better circumstances, would make little sense. "Anti-establishment" ways of thinking might seem appealing now; they certainly appeal to human nature. People respond to "negative values," such as "don't do this" or "don't do that." Religions and ideologies employ this opposition method to influence behavior. For example, of the Ten Commandments, only two are "positive values." The rest declare "thou shalt not do this" or "thou shalt not do that."

Negative values resonate with people far more than positive values. Political campaigns are always "anti-this" or "anti-that." The makings of an idea—and its opposition—are all around us: anti-Americanism, anti-abortion, or anti-discrimination. A successful "anti-anything" campaign needs a good scapegoat, someone or something to blame the problem on.

One surprisingly popular "anti-AIDS" group is called Health Education AIDS Liaison (HEAL). Once considered an odd fringe group founded in the 1980s, HEAL has grown in numbers and has become relatively influential, especially in political debates about AIDS in Africa. The group's mission is to provide "information and support for alternative and holistic approaches to AIDS and related conditions." Chapters are based throughout the United States and Canada, with some local chapters hosting "support" groups.

HEAL has adopted the claims of Duesberg, its battle cry being that people with HIV can stay healthy through "non-toxic, alternative treatments." The group suggests that lifestyle, malnutrition, vaccinations, recreational drugs, illegal street drugs, prescription drugs—including antibiotics and antivirals—sexually transmitted diseases, and psychological and emotional traumas are the true cause of AIDS.

Fringe groups generally rely on scapegoats to fuel their fire. HEAL's pick is the medical establishment and the pharmaceutical industry, which are purportedly in cahoots in a plot to sell "poison" to people for profit. Of course, some lifestyle issues, drugs, and sexually transmitted diseases play a role in good health, but they are not the cause of AIDS. The cause of AIDS is HIV. But if you ask members of HEAL the same question you'll get old research, circular reasoning, and "anti-establishment" philosophies.

Skepticism of established practices can be good. It helps keep some social systems from becoming stagnant. But the danger of cult-like groups like HEAL and other alternative health fanatics, which often prey on the newly diagnosed, is that they twist a few interesting ideas to excess and take advantage of the natural human desire for hope and camaraderie in the face of difficult circumstances.

Having HIV is certainly a difficult circumstance. Learning the news can be incredibly trying. It's natural to have fears and questions about HIV, and it's healthy to have some skepticism about the pharmaceutical industry and the medical community.

However, adopting the philosophies of fanatical groups in place of sound medical advice can have serious and possibly irreparable consequences for your health and well-being. Any extremist group—whether it's on the "alternative" health end of the spectrum or the medical end—should also be viewed with skepticism, especially when the consequences can be detrimental to your health and well being.

IN A SENTENCE:

> *When you hear or learn anything about HIV, consider what's real, what's just an opinion, and what are the true motives of the source.*

living

Alternative Medicine: Mind Over Money?

YEARS AGO, I knew this guy who wrote a column for a neighborhood newspaper. After being diagnosed with HIV, he devoted much of his column to hyping alternative medicine as a valid treatment option for HIV. Over the years, I read his column with an open mind. After all, I was in the same boat: I, too, wondered about the role of alternative medicine.

Ultimately, we took different paths when it came to treating HIV. Over the years, I kept up with his column. He often discussed Chinese herbs and even espoused some "cleansing regimen" that was supposed to eliminate toxins. He claimed it boosted his immune system, which then would fight the virus. With time, however, his health declined, as did his faith in alternative medicine. In his last column, he regretted not having pursued conventional HIV treatment sooner.

It's hard to say what role alternative medicine had in his death. In fact, it's hard to say much at all about alternative medicine because there's usually very little science to back up the claims of the people who profit from this industry. What is a fact is that Americans love alternative medicine, scientifically proven or not.

In this country, individuals pay more out of their own pocket for alternative medicine than they do to see a doctor. One study found that almost half of Americans visit an alternative medicine practitioner during a given year. Like it or not, alternative medicine has a role in living with HIV because, well, Americans keep buying and ingesting everything from St. John's Wort to goat serum.

The terms "alternative," "complementary," and "unconventional" therapy cover several philosophies and approaches. Some approaches are consistent with Western medicine; some are not. Some therapies are so far outside accepted medical practice that they're difficult to evaluate.

Alternative therapy works in some ways

Does alternative medicine work? It depends on what you mean by *work*. If you mean in a capitalistic way, yes, alternative medicine works quite well. The business of alternative medicine is a booming industry, generating some $27 billion a year (to give you some perspective, consider that the pharmaceutical giant Abbott Laboratory generated just under $18 billion in 2002).

Studies have been conducted on why Americans pursue unproven remedies: The top reasons are relief from chronic conditions that include back problems, anxiety, depression, and headaches. For these specific conditions, alternative medicine probably has a role. However, for directly fighting HIV, nothing has yet stood the test of time.

A few studies on alternative medicine and HIV have been published. One study looked at Chinese herbs to treat HIV. The "treatment" was a combination of about a dozen herbs, all of which had been—and still are— highly touted for boosting the immune system and helping with HIV disease. The study was a large, placebo-controlled clinical trial, conducted in five major cities around the United States. According to Daniel S. Berger, M.D., medical director of Northstar Medical Center in Chicago, the results of the trials demonstrated no reduction in HIV and no immune-related benefits for any of the patients in the trial.

"One should be very careful about not getting dragged into the advertising campaigns made by the companies that produce these products," says Berger. "One can go into a health food store and the shelves are full of supplements and vitamins which are bandied in front of the customers, touted as 'good for this' and 'good for that.' You're liable to walk out of the health food store with a shopping cart full of medications. You can spend hundreds or thousands of dollars easily." His message: "Beware."

Consider your motivation for alternative medicine

Having HIV is certainly an understandable reason for anxiety or depression or headaches. So it's no surprise that two-thirds of people with HIV use some form of alternative medicine, including yoga, herbal remedies, massage, megavitamins, folk remedies, energy healing, and homeopathy.

But let's be perfectly clear: Alternative therapy does not improve the course of HIV disease. In the last twenty years, numerous attempts have tried to make the connection that alternative medicine improves HIV. By all accounts, they have failed to show a positive connection. And some alternative therapies are dangerous and can make HIV worse.

If you're considering alternative therapies, first consider your motivations. Are you seeking alternative medicine to fight HIV or to make you feel better in a general sense? The distinction is important. For example, if you're secretly harboring hope that Chinese herbs will raise your T-cell count or lower your viral load, you will be disappointed. Hundreds of thousands of people with AIDS have tried this approach throughout the epidemic.

"I had a lot of patients who spent a huge amount of money doing [alternative] things to extremes and still got very sick," says Berger. He explained that some patients even refused to take conventional HIV treatment and, instead, relied on "high-dose" vitamins and supplements. "They ended up dying," he said.

That was years ago. Today, standard treatments are dramatically improved. There's no good reason—anymore—to look to unproven therapies to keep you healthy. However, if certain forms of alternative medicine—say, yoga, massage, or chiropractic—improve your quality of life and you can afford them, by all means have a field day. Just understand, they don't work for fighting HIV.

For some people, alternative medicine represents a kind of coping strategy, a way to emotionally grapple with a grim situation. "In the old days, when there weren't a lot of [conventional and effective HIV] treatments, patients were desperate, everyone was desperate," says Berger. For combating HIV, Berger said that most of the alternative approaches "don't do much."

Herbal and dietary supplements can be risky

If you like gambling, you'll love herbal medicine. Most herbal or plant-based medicines haven't been properly tested, so they are risky. "Natural" simply means "found in nature." That doesn't mean it's good for you. The poison arsenic is all-natural. If you're taking prescription drugs, be careful about taking herbs or supplements. Some herbs interact with prescription drugs and lead to bad things.

At first, it might make sense that trying to boost your immune system is a way to fight HIV. There's an ongoing war between HIV and the immune system. The immune system can keep HIV in check for many years. But the ongoing battle taxes the immune system.

At some point, the immune system starts to wear down. What it probably needs is a break from the battle and some time to rest and regenerate. It can't rest when HIV is present. The immune systems of some people with HIV eventually burn out.

HIV is a unique virus because it actually feeds on the immune system. When your immune system is activated, HIV is also activated. The virus replicates when T-cells become active. So boosting your immune system is simply giving more food to a hungry virus. It's like fighting a gasoline fire with more gasoline.

Some herbs can hurt

There's no shortage of books, products, and herbal supplements that claim to boost your immune system. For some minor viral infections, alternative therapies might be appropriate in the short term. For HIV, however, boosting your immune system is probably not a good long-term strategy.

"Some of these [alternative] medications can cause allergic reactions," says Berger. "Also, they can cause diarrhea, which reduces the absorption of [conventional HIV] medications." This, he said, can cause the HIV medications to fail. "So taking herbs or supplements may not be harmless."

If you are taking any medicine—HIV treatment included—you should know about potential interactions between the drugs and herbs. Supplements and herbs are not regulated by the Food and Drug Administration because they are considered food products and nutritional adjuncts, not drugs. As such, the interactions of many alternative products and HIV medicines have not been well studied.

A few herbs to watch out for:

ECHINACEA
Sometimes called Purple Coneflower, Echinacea is a flowering plant once used by Native Americans. Several interesting studies in Europe have examined Echinacea. Americans annually spend about $300 million on the herb, according to the National Institutes of Health. It's one of the most

frequently sold herbs, primarily to treat colds and flu by stimulating the immune system.

Echinacea is controversial for people with HIV. Some doctors believe that, since HIV feeds on the immune system, it's not wise to stimulate the immune system on a regular basis. Other doctors believe that the immune system is already overactive from fighting HIV and Echinacea may add more stress. There is no published research to document dangerous results from the use of Echinacea by people with HIV. Some researchers believe that short-term use (up to two weeks) to treat colds or flu doesn't pose any serious risks.

In a study conducted in 2002, Echinacea showed no detectable benefit or harm when given to a small group of people without HIV who were suffering from cold symptoms, such as sore throats and stuffy noses. However, the author of the study said anecdotal reports about Echinacea's benefits were "difficult to ignore" despite this discouraging research. At least two large studies in Germany concluded the herb was safe and effective for treating cold symptoms.

St. John's Wort

Do not use St. John's Wort if you're taking anti-HIV drugs. St. John's Wort is a plant product used to relieve mild depression. It can cause serious problems when mixed with other medicines, including the anti-HIV drug indinavir (Crixivan). Bad reactions also have been reported in people who combine it with antidepressants. How it helps depression is unclear, but the way it works may be similar to that of pharmaceutical drugs. Be sure to tell your doctor if you're taking St. John's Wort, or at least ask your doctor about potential drug interactions.

Garlic Supplements

Potentially harmful side effects have been reported when garlic supplements were taken in conjunction with the anti-HIV drug saquinavir (Fortovase). Be cautious about using garlic supplements during HIV therapy.

Consult an HIV-experienced professional before taking herbs or supplements

How do you make reasonable decisions about herbs and supple-ments? Daniel S. Berger, M.D., notes that there are few options. "If your physician happens to be savvy, or somewhat knowledgeable regarding supplements, vitamins, and minerals, you should definitely consult with your physician. If your physician isn't, then consult with a nutritionist that's HIV-knowledgeable."

Berger cautions people not to pursue the herbal or supplement route on their own. "A lot of articles and information on the Internet are done by publicists or people who are trying to increase revenue for companies that are selling the products." Just because information is on the Internet, doesn't make it valid.

Put aside the question of the effectiveness of alternative medicine. A more important question is: How are you going to pay for it? Except for chiropractic and sometimes acupuncture, chances are good that it's not covered by health insurance. If committing to a course of some herb or supplement, don't forget you'll be paying for it over the long haul. Small expenses begin to add up when $35 a month becomes $420 a year.

Alternative medicine helps the mind

If you're looking for ways to reduce stress, anxiety, or depression—and the symptoms that stem from these underlying conditions—chances are much better you'll find some alternative medicines beneficial.

YOGA

Yoga is a general term for several spiritual practices that are designed to help people achieve a "higher consciousness" and liberation from suffering. The basic concept behind yoga is that one can gain a better perspective by practicing certain behaviors. Hatha is the most popular type of yoga in the United States and it emphasizes physical control and postures. Yoga has been shown to help with depression, anxiety, heart disease, high blood pressure, headaches, and some forms of chronic pain. It has not been shown to have a direct impact on HIV.

It's hard to explain the benefits of yoga. Some people say it reduces stress by stretching tense muscles and relaxing tight spines. Other people suggest that the mental concentration required by yoga allows them to forget about the worries of daily life. Most people just say they feel better after doing yoga.

A good place to start yoga is in a group class. Most AIDS services organizations can direct you to a reputable yoga class or instructor. Often, such classes are free to people with HIV. If you're new to yoga, take a beginner's class. You'll be surprised how physically demanding it can be.

• • •

MASSAGE

Who doesn't feel better after a good massage? There's some evidence that speaks to the reparative qualities of massage. But if you've ever had a good, or at least an enthusiastic massage, then you shouldn't need to be convinced about the merits of massage. At its simplest, massage gives the feeling of general relaxation, as tight muscles are pulled and stretched. Massage styles can range from gentle rocking to intense deep-tissue kneading.

There's an aspect to massage that extends beyond simple pushing and pulling of muscles. Some people say the value-added benefit to massage therapy is the human element. They say some of the potency of massage comes from the instinctual desire to touch and be touched. Babies die without the coddling of an adult. So it makes intuitive sense that expressions of affection such as touching, rubbing, holding, and squeezing are good, not just for the body, but for the soul.

CHIROPRACTIC

Chiropractic medicine attempts to restore normal function of the body by manipulation and treatment of the body structures, especially the back. Through manipulation, chiropractors may be able to relieve joint stiffness and pain. Studies have unequivocally shown chiropractic to be effective for acute lower back pain.

MEDITATION

Meditation uses deep breathing or other techniques to tune out the day-to-day mental chatter and thereby lower anxiety and stress. Some research has shown that meditation can bring about a lowering of heart rate, a decrease in respiration, a decrease in levels of a stress hormone called cortisol, and an increase in brain waves associated with relaxation. Some physicians, therapists, and healthcare workers recommend meditation as a way to relax.

ACUPUNCTURE

This therapy involves the painless insertion of thin needles into the skin to balance the body's flow of energy, referred to as **qi** ("chee"). Acupuncture is sometimes used to relieve neuropathy, fatigue, anxiety, and pain. Acupuncture has been studied for a specific type of pain called HIV-related peripheral neuropathy. It was shown to be no more effective than placebo.

IN A SENTENCE:

> *Herbs and supplements do not work for treating HIV, but some forms of alternative medicine help with symptoms of anxiety and depression.*

learning

T-Cell Counts and Viral Load Tests

THERE ARE two kinds of blood tests worth paying attention to:

○ HIV viral load
○ CD4+ cell count (T-cell count)

Consider these tests, also known as **surrogate markers,** as important as a compass and the North Star were to ancient sailors. The results of these two tests will greatly influence your treatment options.

The viral load test measures *how fast* HIV disease is progressing, and the T-cell count reflects *how far* HIV disease has progressed. In general, it's a good thing when your T-cell count is high and your viral load is low or undetectable. On the other hand, it's a bad thing when your T-cell counts are low or your viral load is high.

Imagine a car. Think of your T-cells as the gasoline in the car. The faster you drive, the faster you run out of gas. However, if you start out with a full tank of gas, driving for a long time is no problem. In the same way, if your T-cells are high, living a long time is a given.

• • •

Using this example, your viral load is like the speed of the car. The higher the viral load, the faster the disease is progressing. If your viral load is high, it's like you're speeding—and when you run out of gas will depend on what's in your tank. If you're speeding and your T-cells are higher, you've got a ways to go. If you're speeding and your T-cells are low, you're asking for trouble.

	High	**Low**
T-cells:	good	bad
Viral Load:	bad	good

T-cells are a barometer of your immune system

T-cells are special cells found in your blood. They make up the biggest part of your immune system. Without T-cells, your immune system couldn't fight the viruses, bacteria, and fungi that constantly invade the body. In a twist of fate, T-cells are the most popular target for HIV. The virus infects the very cell designed to fight it.

In healthy people without HIV, the CD4+ T-cell count is generally somewhere between 500 and 1,200 cells per cubic millimeter of blood. A cubic millimeter is equal to about one drop of blood. This measurement is often shortened to ml or mL. A T-cell count of 450 might be written as CD4 = 450 ml.

In the absence of anti-HIV treatment, the T-cell count decreases an average of about 50 to 100 cells each year. The critical threshold for your T-cells is around 200. At that point, it seems, the body becomes especially vulnerable to infections.

T-CELLS 500 OR ABOVE—HIGH

If your T-cells are in this range, it means that HIV has done minimal damage to your immune system.

T-CELLS 499 TO 200—MID-RANGE

A count in this range means that HIV has already caused a mild to moderate amount of damage to your immune system.

T-CELLS 199 TO 0—LOW

If your count falls in this range, it means that HIV has done severe damage to your immune system. If your count falls in this range, you should be taking special antibiotics to prevent a certain type of pneumonia often referred to simply as **PCP**.

How should you feel about your T-cell count?

There are some important things to know about these T-cell counts. A single T-cell count does not mean as much as several T-cells counts taken over time. For example, it's impossible to tell from a single test if your T-cells are rising or falling. Also, T-cell counts naturally fluctuate somewhat. They can be lower if you have a cold or flu when you take the test or higher if your immune system is activated for some reason. The best indicator of your immune system is the overall trend of your T-cell counts over time.

Still, if your T-cell count is lower than you hoped it would be, you're bound to be disappointed. It's all too easy to fixate on a low T-cell count. The news might even lead you to feel nervous or anxious. At first, you may seem okay when hearing that your T-cells are low. But later, you might feel overwhelmed, you might cry, or even find yourself seeking distractions like drugs or alcohol.

There's no one-size-fits-all way of responding to your first T-cell count. In general, if your T-cells are in the high range, you should feel good that you've caught your HIV earlier, before it had a chance to cause much damage. If your T-cells are in the middle range, don't panic. But pay attention by closely monitoring your counts. If your T-cells are low, you should be concerned and you should be taking medications to prevent certain opportunistic infections.

Whatever your T-cell count, it's still only half the picture. The T-cell count can tell you how much damage has already been done to your immune system. It cannot tell you how quickly the damage is being done. The second part of the equation is the HIV viral load.

Viral load is a snapshot of the virus

Before HIV viral load testing was available, doctors and researchers thought the virus stayed dormant for several years after initial infection. However, researchers used viral load testing to learn that, in fact, the immune system and virus are locked in a fierce battle from day one.

Generally speaking, viral load testing employs a technology that finds and amplifies small particles of **DNA**. HIV doesn't have DNA but rather a similar material called **RNA**. The HIV viral load test finds bits of RNA that come from HIV. The test then amplifies the RNA so that it can be measured. The RNA would be impossible to measure unless it was amplified.

There are two main types of viral load tests available: **PCR** and **bDNA**. The abbreviation PCR stands for polymerase chain reaction, and bDNA stands for branched-chain DNA.

The tests are sometimes used for different stages of HIV disease. PCR is the most sensitive and can detect very low levels of virus in the blood, but the bDNA test has been shown to be the most accurate in measuring high levels of virus. Keep in mind that every test has some level of error.

Viral load seems to be a good predictor of disease progression. Viral load tests use the word "copies" to refer to the unit of measurement. For example, a person may get a viral load result of 60,000 copies. Keep in mind that viral copies are measured exponentially. This is different than your T-cell count, which is measured in a linear way, more like the gasoline gauge on your car. For example, the difference between 60,000 and 6,000 is 10 times less or 90 percent less. The difference between 60,000 copies and 60 copies is 100 times less or 99 percent less.

Sometimes, doctors will refer to "**log** drops" in viral load. A log drop basically means a 90 percent reduction in the level of virus. So, the difference between 60,000 and 6,000 is a one-log drop. The difference between 60,000 and 600 is a two-log drop. A one-log reduction from 150,000 copies to 15,000 copies is the same thing as, say, a one-log reduction from 50,000 to 5,000 copies. Don't worry if this doesn't make a lot of sense right now.

For viral loads, less is better

A high viral load is bad. It literally means that there's more virus in your blood and that the disease is progressing quickly. A low viral load is considered a good thing. It means there's less virus in your blood and the disease is progressing more slowly. Most sensitive viral load tests can measure down to 50 copies of virus. If there are 49 copies, the result will be "undetectable." Clearly, the virus is not gone, it's just below what the test can detect.

People with viral load levels over 100,000 copies are 10 times more likely to get sick over the next five years as compared to those with levels below 100,000 copies. Furthermore, people with constant viral load levels below 10,000 seem to have a much lower risk of disease progression. But it doesn't mean that the disease won't progress, it only means that the chance of its progressing is lower.

HIV Viral Load

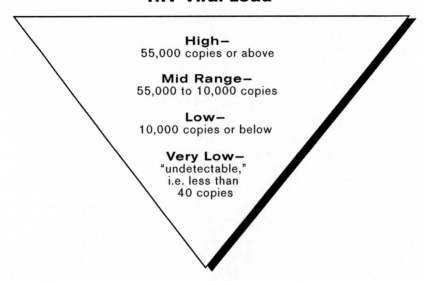

High—
55,000 copies or above

Mid Range—
55,000 to 10,000 copies

Low—
10,000 copies or below

Very Low—
"undetectable,"
i.e. less than
40 copies

In the normal progression of HIV disease, viral levels tend to rise slowly. As in the case of T-cell counts, a viral load test can vary. Other infections can cause a temporary increase in HIV viral levels. Some doctors may take two viral load tests, about two to four weeks apart, to establish a baseline level. Tests can vary slightly in their results, so if you're using a particular test you should continue to use the same test.

T-cell plus viral load equals immune strength

Using both T-cell counts and viral load testing gives you and your doctor a more complete picture of your health and the status of your immune system. While T-cell counts reflect your body's firepower for fighting disease, viral load tests indicate the activity of the virus. So what do these tests mean for your life right now? Here's a chart to help you organize your thoughts:

T-cells + Viral Load	Possible Meanings
High + Low	Your immune system is in good shape and the virus seems to be suppressed for some reason. Celebrate, this is great news. Monitor your T-cells and viral load every 3-4 months.
High + High	Your immune system is still in good shape, but it's not likely to stay that way. Since the virus is active, your immune system is likely to break down soon.
Low + Low	In this case, damage has been done in the past, but the virus is currently being held in check.
Low + High	Not good. Your immune system is damaged and your body is vulnerable to other infections. The virus is replicating quickly, further depleting your immune system.

IN A SENTENCE:

A viral load test measures how fast HIV disease is progressing and a T-cell count reflects how far HIV disease has progressed.

FIRST-MONTH MILESTONE

By the end of the first month, you're beginning to get a handle on how to cope with many issues involved with having HIV:

○ YOU KNOW WHY IT'S IMPORTANT TO SHOP AROUND BEFORE CHOOSING AN HIV DOCTOR, AND HOW TO MAKE THE MOST OF YOUR LIMITED TIME WITH THAT PERSON, AND HOW HIV AFFECTS THE IMMUNE SYSTEM.

○ YOU UNDERSTAND THAT TELLING OTHER PEOPLE ABOUT YOUR HIV STATUS IS ALWAYS YOUR OWN DECISION, ONE THAT SHOULD BE CAREFULLY CONSIDERED BEFOREHAND.

○ WHEN YOU HEAR OR LEARN ANYTHING ABOUT HIV, YOU KNOW TO CONSIDER WHAT'S REAL, WHAT'S JUST AN OPINION, AND WHAT'S THE TRUE MOTIVE OF THE SOURCE OF INFORMATION.

○ YOU HAVE LEARNED THAT HERBS AND SUPPLEMENTS DO NOT WORK FOR TREATING HIV, BUT SOME FORMS OF ALTERNATIVE MEDICINE CAN HELP WITH ANXIETY AND DEPRESSION.

○ YOU HAVE BEEN INTRODUCED TO THE MEANING OF A VIRAL LOAD TEST, WHICH MEASURES HOW FAST HIV DISEASE IS PROGRESSING, AND TO THE MEANING OF A T-CELL COUNT, WHICH REFLECTS HOW FAR HIV DISEASE HAS PROGRESSED.

Dating and Sex

DATING ISN'T easy. Even in the best of circumstances, courtship is complicated. Inevitably, the interaction is charged with emotions and expectations. Introduce the wild card of HIV, and the stakes get raised. And for couples where only one person has HIV, the delicate ritual is even more fragile.

Some relationships between HIV-positives and negatives survive and some don't. Many just never happen to begin with. The pairing of opposites is possible, but it takes work—plenty of work. Now that you know you have HIV, the search for Mr. or Ms. Right may seem impossible. You might have fears of rejection. You might feel like a biohazard or damaged goods.

Many people may choose to shut down or simply take themselves off the market, opting out of dating altogether. These are normal responses, especially early on after an HIV diagnosis. These feelings usually subside with time.

Ultimately, HIV shouldn't deter you from the pursuit of romance. Plenty of HIV-positive people go on to have successful relationships, marriages, and even families. You may not be ready to get involved with another person right away, but it's a relief to know it is possible.

• • •

Issues can emerge for both parties

In the dating world, problems are likely to come up for you and your partner. The fear of contagion is quite real for both partners. For the HIV-negative person, the issue is how to avoid becoming infected. For the positive partner, the fear is of giving the virus to the other person— something that might seem unforgivable. For many HIV-positive people, a little voice inside their head constantly monitors and restricts their every movement.

It's possible to test the dating waters with other HIV-positive people. However, many people are perfectly comfortable dating someone who is HIV-negative. Either way, finding the right time to disclose the news isn't easy. Furthermore, people have very different thoughts on the matter.

Rosetta M., an HIV educator from Buffalo, New York, is the kind of person who discloses her HIV status sooner rather than later. "I wanted to find out who would stand and who would fall away," says Rosetta M. "I realized I didn't need everybody, but I needed a few 'somebodies.' The only way to find them was to let them know who I was. HIV is part of who I am."

Not everyone is as forthcoming. Some people choose to disclose their HIV status after having sex. "I always have safe sex, so it wasn't like I put anyone in danger," says Alan G. "But I told [the person whom I had sex with] over the phone and he freaked. Subsequent phone calls from the guy were threatening. I didn't know what to do. The last time we spoke, I listened to his frustrations and analyzed them for my own. I'm still not sure who to tell on the first date. Sometimes I do, sometimes I don't."

"I couldn't imagine even accepting a date from a person who didn't know I was HIV-positive," says Rosetta. "I let a lot of people know. I knew that when people asked me out, they already knew." In fact, Rosetta is now married to a man who is HIV-negative. "We made eye contact for six months. Then we started to date. Within four months, he realized what an awesome person I was and wanted to marry me."

It always takes two to tango. From the perspective of someone who's HIV-negative, dating a person who is positive may be too scary. There's no shortage of stories about people who were rejected because of their HIV status. But there are also a few success stories.

"My roommate kept telling me about a guy who I would really like, but that I shouldn't go out with him because he suspected that the guy was HIV positive," says Brian K., who is HIV-negative. "Well, I did meet him and we fell in love. He is now my partner. He told me on our second date, before we had a chance to have sex. It didn't hinder my dating him at all. We have been together now for four years. He is a wonderful man."

Steven G. tells a similar story. "My partner worries about getting HIV from me, but ultimately he overlooks it," he says. "I guess he must think I'm worth the sacrifice."

Disclosure Tactics

NOT SURE how to break the HIV news to a date? Here are some personal accounts of how to handle disclosure:

○ I have always told on the first date, sitting across from the person, looking them in their face. Not on the phone, where rejection comes easily. Not in a bar, where alcohol and music can prevent any real conversation. First date, face to face. If he rejects me, he would have had to do so the adult way, the brave way, looking at me, having talked to me and gotten to know me.

○ I don't disclose a thing about HIV until I get to trust the person. I try to get a sense if the person is okay with HIV stuff or not. I drop a hint by saying a good friend of mine has AIDS. I carefully watch how he responds to the hint. You'd be surprised at what you can learn from body language.

○ I make no big secret of my status. It's part of who I am. It's not the only part, so I don't put it in front of my name. But I couldn't imagine a first date going by without this disclosure. At the end of the day, you have to look at yourself in the mirror.

○ I always tell before I'm asked. I indicate my HIV status before I ask others.

Put your emotions aside when thinking about sex

Many people with HIV worry about infecting others. For some people, these worries may even escalate to intense conflict or anxiety. The best way to deal with these concerns is to learn how HIV is transmitted and be honest with yourself about your own sexual behavior.

You might feel awkward or a little guilty when thinking about sex. In fact, you may find yourself wanting to avoid the topic altogether. While reading the remainder of this chapter, put aside your emotions about sex. Emotions don't transmit HIV, specific sexual behaviors do. For now, consider how these behaviors might affect other people. Deal with your emotions about sex later.

A word of caution about discussing sex: Be very selective about the people in whom you confide. Emotions, personal and religious biases, and even outright hostility can surface in people, even in those who may be close to you. Sex and morality are hot-button issues with almost everyone.

People have vastly different opinions about sex and HIV. I've had many acquaintances, some friends, and even professional counselors react negatively or disapprovingly to the idea that HIV-positive people should pursue sex. Make no apologies for wanting a full sex life, just be cautious about the people with whom you discuss the topic.

There will always be isolated stories about someone who apparently got HIV in some obscure way. Don't give in to this sensationalism. The bottom line is that, in terms of sex, the primary way for you to pass HIV is through blood or semen that gets inside another person. This can happen through the anus (a.k.a. rectum) or vagina. It is very unlikely, but still possible, to pass the virus through genital-to-mouth contact.

The difference between "safe sex" and "safer sex" is just a letter

It's impossible to precisely define "safe" and "unsafe" sexual behavior. In reality, there's only gray area—a continuum of choices—between the two extremes. Among the politically correct crowd, the term *safe sex* is supposed to be a no-no. The correct term to use is *safer sex*. But regular people don't always speak in politically correct terms. So, from here on, I'll refer to *safer* sex as *safe* sex because that's the way we all speak in normal conversations and the difference is only the words, not their meanings. After you understand the realities of how HIV is transmitted, you'll need to weigh the risks and benefits to yourself and to your potential sex partners.

Masturbation is safe sex

Of course, masturbation is the act of stimulating your own genitals using your own hands, or other objects, often to the point of orgasm. It's normal and healthy, despite various claims to the contrary. Most everyone masturbates, whether or not they admit to it.

Solo masturbation—without physical contact with another person—is one of the only sexual activities that carries no risk of giving or getting sexually transmitted diseases, including HIV.

The Facts:

HIV LIVES IN:
blood
semen (commonly called "cum")
pre-cum (fluid that drips from the penis during arousal)
vaginal fluids
menstrual blood (blood from a woman's period)
breast milk

YOU CANNOT GET HIV THROUGH:
saliva
sweat
urine
feces (as long as blood is not present)
skin-to-skin contact (as long as there are no cuts, abrasions, or sores)

If you have the virus, solo masturbation is a great way of getting sexual pleasure without all the complications that come with another person. In fact, some people masturbate simply to relieve stress or boredom. Whatever the reason, masturbating is completely safe.

Some people carry around subconscious messages from religious backgrounds or from parents that lead to guilt or uncomfortable feelings about masturbating. But don't let that stop you.

For men, using a lubricant during masturbation can help prevent soreness to the penis. There are lots of great "lubes" on the market; look for those that are water-based since they wash off the body easily (and are safe to use with latex condoms). Hand lotion or Vaseline can be used to masturbate, but remember, these contain oils that can damage condoms.

Semen can transmit HIV, so be aware of where your semen ends up. After ejaculation, there will probably be semen on your genitals or your hands. Most guys clean up with a towel, napkin, or even clothing. Both men and women should avoid sharing dildos or sex toys with other people as small amounts of blood, semen, or vaginal secretions might remain on them. If other people use the same dildo or toys as you, it's unlikely but still possible to transmit HIV this way. If you do share toys, wash them well with warm soapy water.

Is getting "head" safe?

Can you pass HIV to another person through oral contact or oral sex? It is possible, but very unlikely. A study published in 2002 found that getting HIV from oral contact with someone's penis is a very rare event. The study looked at men who have sex with men, who exclusively performed oral sex as the person who was "giving head." Twenty-eight percent of the men studied knew their partner had HIV and of those, 35 percent reported getting semen in their mouths. None of the men in the study tested positive for HIV.

On the other hand, another recent study funded by the Centers for Disease Control and Prevention (CDC) found that 7.8 percent of recently infected men who have sex with men were "probably infected through oral sex." One problem with this study, however, was that some of the men who became infected had also engaged in other risky behaviors, so it was hard to identify the real cause. Nearly half of the men who did test HIV-positive reported having oral problems, such as occasional bleeding gums.

If someone engages in oral contact with your penis, or gives you a "blow job," here are some things you can do to reduce the risk to other people:

○ avoid being sucked if you have sores or cuts on your penis
○ avoid being sucked if your partner has bleeding gums, sores, or cuts in his or her mouth
○ avoid ejaculating (cumming) in the other person's mouth

Your mouth and someone's penis

If you suck another person's penis, there is very little chance that HIV can get out of your body. There is wide agreement that "giving head" poses an extremely low risk of passing the virus to another person. In other words, don't worry much about giving the virus to someone if *you* give a blow job. A bigger concern for you is catching additional sexually transmitted diseases (the last part of this section offers more details on condoms).

Someone's mouth and your vagina

Mouth-to-vagina contact is often referred to as "going down," "eating out," or "eating pussy." A less common term is **cunnilingus**. It's a form of oral sex that involves the stimulation of the vagina by the mouth and tongue, and it's quite common.

If you have HIV and someone's mouth comes into contact with your vagina, the potential risk to that person may come from the discharge of your vaginal secretions, or your menstrual blood, into the mouth of another person.

Studies on the risks of cunnilingus are rare. There are only a few documented cases by the CDC that demonstrate HIV transmission to a person performing oral contact on a woman. This is the best evidence that the risk of transmission through cunnilingus is very low.

It's often suggested that women with HIV use a specially-designed-for-cunnilingus latex barrier called a **dental dam**, or even plastic food wrap (such as Saran Wrap). However, given the potentially low risk of passing HIV by cunnilingus, and the lack of research to document the success of dental dams, most women find them, well, ridiculous.

Someone's mouth and your butt

The act of stimulating the anus by the mouth and tongue is called **anilingus** or more commonly "rimming." The anus has nerve endings in the pelvic region and many people find stimulation to be sexually arousing.

The CDC has clearly stated that fecal matter, in the absence of blood, is not considered to be a bodily fluid that transmits HIV and, therefore, poses minimal risk for transmitting the virus. A potential source of risk for the person who is rimming you would be from very small amounts of blood that may be present in or around your anus. Anal bleeding can occur by prior sexual penetration.

Your mouth and someone's butt

If you "eat" someone's butt (in other words, you do the rimming), there is very little chance that HIV can get out of your body and into theirs. This behavior poses an extremely low risk of passing the virus to another person.

Rimming another person, however, leaves you susceptible to catching additional sexually transmitted diseases. There's considerable risk for contracting hepatitis A and hepatitis B, parasites or "bugs," and a host of other infections.

Urine

Urine does not transmit HIV. Even if the urine contained small amounts of blood, the urine itself would kill the virus.

Your penis and someone's vagina

If you have HIV and you insert your penis in someone's vagina, it's quite possible that you can transmit the virus. In fact, it's the most common way the virus is transmitted in the world. HIV can live in blood, semen, and pre-cum.

The vagina is relatively fragile compared with the mouth. The lining of the vagina can tear and possibly allow HIV to enter a women's body. Tiny cuts or sores inside a vagina can be small or invisible. The virus can pass through the mucous membranes that line the vagina and get inside the woman with whom you're having sex.

For many years, it was believed that an ingredient that was often used in lubricants called **nonoxynol-9** or N-9 might prevent HIV during sexual intercourse. The CDC has declared that N-9 gel does not prevent HIV. In fact, using the N-9 during anal or vaginal intercourse may actually increase the chances that HIV will be transmitted. Some brands of lubricated condoms contain N-9—don't use them.

If you have HIV and you insert your penis into someone's vagina without wearing a latex condom, you are putting that person at a high risk for contracting HIV. Withdrawing your penis before ejaculation is not sufficient protection because of the presence of HIV in pre-cum. The vagina is more susceptible (especially when compared with the mouth), and may allow the virus to get into your partner's bloodstream. You can greatly reduce the risk to your partner by using a latex condom from start to finish (the last part of this section offers more details on condoms).

Someone's penis and your vagina

In general, men are at lower risk of getting HIV from vaginal fluids or menstrual blood. The potential risk comes from vaginal fluid or menstrual blood that comes in contact with the opening of the penis. In fact, some studies have found that, during vaginal intercourse without a condom, a woman with HIV is half as likely to transmit the virus to a man than the other way around. However, the risk increases somewhat if the man has a sore patch of skin on his penis.

If someone comes in contact with your blood during sex, this increases the risk of passing the virus. For example, there may be blood in the vagina if intercourse occurs during a woman's period. You can greatly reduce the risk to your partner by using a latex condom from start to finish (the last part of this section offers more details on condoms).

Someone's penis and your butt

There's some controversy about the risks of anal sex or anal-penis contact. If your anus is penetrated by someone's penis—without a condom—the risk of your passing HIV to someone else is minimal, at least when compared with other sexual acts.

The potential risk comes from small, sometimes invisible amounts of blood that come in contact with the opening of the penis or with sore patches of skin on the penis. If someone comes in contact with your blood during sex, this increases the risk of passing the virus. For example, there may be blood in or around your anus if intercourse occurred beforehand. You can greatly reduce the risk to your partner by having that person use a latex condom from start to finish (see the next section of this chapter for details on condoms).

When it comes to anal sex or anal-penis contact without a condom, there is some potential risk to you. This risk comes from the possibility of someone infecting you with a different strain of HIV. In fact, researchers have documented a case of an individual who was infected with a second strain of HIV, one that was more difficult to control.

Your penis and someone's butt

In the continuum between low and high risk, you inserting your penis in someone's anus carries the highest risk for that person. The lining of the anus is even more delicate than the lining of the vagina or the mouth. So it is much more likely to get small cuts or abrasions during sexual contact. Because of this, as well the mucous membranes that line the anus, anal intercourse is a very efficient way to pass the virus.

You can greatly reduce the risk to your partner by using a latex condom from start to finish (see the next section of this chapter for details on condoms). Even if you use a condom, the risk to another person is still relatively higher when compared to oral sex.

Let's be clear, it doesn't matter if you're straight or gay. In fact, researchers have examined the risk for heterosexual HIV transmission to women by HIV-positive men. In couples that engaged in both anal and vaginal intercourse, 62 percent of the cases where HIV transmission occurred were due to anal contact. The researchers reported that the risk for anal contact was 10 times higher than the risk for vaginal contact.

For men who have sex with men, a large study found that about 10 percent got HIV if they engaged in "receptive anal intercourse" (that is, they were the "bottom" partner) with at least two different people over the course of six months. The researchers concluded that "receptive anal intercourse was the only significant risk factor" for getting HIV. This—and many other studies—clearly demonstrate that anal sex without a condom carries the highest risk.

If you have HIV and you insert your penis into someone's anus—without wearing a condom—you are putting your partner at a very high risk for contracting HIV. Withdrawing your penis before ejaculation is not sufficient protection, since pre-cum also contains HIV.

Barebacking happens mostly in the news

There's been a lot of media hype and debate among public health officials about a phenomenon called **barebacking**. The term is defined as intentionally seeking out and engaging in anal intercourse without a condom, whether it's by the "insertive" (top) participant or the "receptive" (bottom) participant. The intentional part distinguishes barebacking from poor planning or spontaneous decisions about not using condoms.

The issue got attention in the gay community, where reports surfaced of a new "subculture" of gay men—mostly HIV-positive—who threw parties, visited sex clubs, and adopted an identity based on the thrill of having sex without condoms. The issue prompted emotional and contentious debates, especially as some speculated that as many as 65 percent of gay men were barebacking.

As it turned out, the issue may have been overblown. In 2002, the CDC announced the results of a large study the incidence of barebacking to be only 14 percent. Although the study found that 22 percent of HIV-positive men acknowledged barebacking—versus 10 percent for the HIV-negative group—the majority of HIV-positive men engaged in this activity with other HIV-positive men. Researchers concluded that there is a relatively small number of "hard-core barebackers." Primary motivators included enhanced physical stimulation and emotional connectedness.

An unfortunate fallout from the bareback phenomenon is the public perception of HIV-positive men as irresponsible. As such, health officials have responded with programs and media campaigns that call for men with HIV to always disclose their HIV status to potential sex partners.

At the same time, new studies confirmed that about half the people in the United States who have HIV are not aware of their own infection. Public health campaigns, however, call for full disclosure of HIV status—an impossible goal if you don't know you have the virus. The most prudent approach for everyone is to practice safe sex as often as possible rather than relying on others to reveal their HIV status. If you have HIV, ultimately what matters is what you do, not what you say.

Using condoms is like wearing seat belts in a car

It would be ideal if everyone used condoms, but, let's be real, not everybody does. If you already have HIV, all the rhetoric you see or hear about wearing condoms to prevent HIV suddenly loses its punch. You've probably been told dozens of times to use condoms for vaginal and anal sex so I won't repeat it.

I will, however, offer you some straightforward reasons on why you should use latex condoms as often as possible:

○ Condoms offer you protection from a long list of nasty STDs that can damage your immune system and may shorten your life.

○ Condoms can greatly reduce your chance of getting or giving genital herpes or genital warts (the next section of this chapter offers more details on herpes and warts). While condoms don't entirely prevent the transmission of these diseases, they spin the odds in your favor. There are many strains of both herpes and warts. Even if you already have one strain, you can still get another.

○ Condoms can prevent you from getting strains of HIV that may be worse than the one you already have. This has been documented (it's called "super-infection" and you don't want it). You're in this for the long haul, so keeping out unwanted strains of HIV will help you preserve your health in the years to come.

○ Condoms may help you avoid awkward or even illegal situations. You may be too fearful to disclose your HIV status to others—but you can wear a condom without disclosing your status or arousing suspicion in others. Remember, when it comes to sex, what matters most is not what you say, but what you do.

Practice using condoms alone at first

Let's face it, using condoms can be awkward, especially when you're not completely familiar with them. One way to get a "feel" for condoms is to

How to Put on a Condom

STUDIES HAVE shown that condoms break less than 2 percent of the time. Most of the breakage is due to incorrect use, rather than poor condom quality. In case no one has told you how to properly wear a condom, here's a reminder:

1. First off, don't store condoms in a glove compartment or in your wallet; heat and sunlight may damage them. Don't use old condoms or ones that are beyond their expiration date. Don't open them with your teeth and be mindful of fingernails. They can be torn.

2. Most condoms have a small pouch at the tip designed to catch the semen. Put a few drops of water-based lube inside the tip. Force the air from the pouch at the tip of the condom by squeezing it.

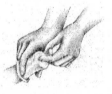

3. Put the condom on after the penis is hard. Squeeze the tip of the condom to leave some extra space; but ensure that no air is trapped in the tip. (The water-based lube should fill the space.) Roll the rest down the shaft of the penis. When fully unrolled, the condom should extend almost to the base of the penis.

4. If the penis has a foreskin, put the condom on with the foreskin pushed back. Once the shaft is covered, push the foreskin forward (toward the tip). This lets the foreskin move without breaking the condom.

5. Put more water-based lube on the outside of the condom.

6. After ejaculation, the condom should be removed carefully to prevent semen from spilling out. To do this, the penis is withdrawn while holding the condom securely to the penis (so it doesn't get left behind). After removal, dispose of the condom and don't reuse it.

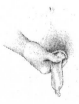

collect several different kinds of them first. Then, try masturbating with them. You'll probably find a specific brand that fits best. Save the package so you remember what brand you'll want to use regularly. Here are some important tips to keep in mind:

- ○ Using oil-based lubricants can weaken latex, causing the condom to break. In addition, condoms can be weakened by exposure to heat or sunlight, or by age. Teeth or fingernails can also tear them.
- ○ Different types and brands of condoms are available from almost any drug store. Remember, only latex condoms stop HIV. Natural membrane ("skin" or "lambskin") condoms are designed to stop pregnancy, not HIV, so don't use them. Female condoms are also available, but their usefulness for HIV has not been well studied.
- ○ Some condoms come with lubrication ("pre-lubed"), others don't. Either way, do not use hand lotion, moisturizer, cold creams, Vaseline, baby oil, mineral oil, vegetable oil, Crisco, or any other products that contain oils. Oils can damage condoms and cause them to break.
- ○ When using condoms, use only water-based lubes. Some water-based lubes include Astroglide, KY, Probe, and Wet. An easy way to tell the difference between oil- and water-based lubes is how they "bead" water. If you're not sure, read the label. If you're still not sure, don't use it.
- ○ For condoms to provide maximum protection, they must be used correctly. Use a new condom each time you engage in sex. Do not use a condom more than once.

IN A SENTENCE:

Understand that only certain sexual behaviors can transmit HIV and such behaviors can affect your health and the health of other people.

learning

Herpes and HPV

YOU WANT to stay as healthy as possible for as long as possible. Right? There's no single "thing" you can do to achieve this goal—except for one: Make better choices over time. Each choice you make—or don't make—will have some effect down the road. Making choices about your health today will affect your health in future. You probably wish you could go back in time and "undo" HIV. All you can do is make better choices now.

Thinking about the "long term" may seem strange to you because of the uncertainties of HIV. However, given all the new HIV treatments and the ones coming down the pipeline, thinking about the future becomes even more important. Your behavior today, this week, and this month can directly affect your health, say, a year from now, five years from now, or twenty years from now.

People with HIV sometimes forget about the long term. Two of the biggest health issues facing people with HIV are two viruses that people rarely talk about: herpes and warts (**HPV**). You probably already know that "cold sores" or blisters on your lips, face, and genitals are caused by a virus. This virus makes HIV worse, and HIV makes the herpes virus worse. Genital warts are also caused by a virus, although it's different from both HIV and herpes. Genital warts in people with HIV are usually worse than in those without HIV. Even more troubling is that warts can cause cancer, especially in people with HIV.

But don't let yourself get freaked out about herpes or warts. If you don't have them already, you can prevent them both. If you suspect you have either herpes or warts, you can treat them or keep them in check, which will help with your HIV. Either way, you will be better off by having a basic understanding of these common viruses. This way, you'll make better choices now and in the years to come.

Genital herpes is extremely common

Herpes is the most common **sexually transmitted disease (STD)** among people with HIV. Even among the general population, about one in five is infected with the virus that causes genital herpes, and the prevalence has jumped 30 percent since the late 1970s. Other STDs such as gonorrhea, syphilis, and chlamydia are legally required to be reported to the CDC, and public health officials try to find and treat people who may have been exposed. This type of tracking and treatment is not the case with herpes.

There are many different types of viruses within the *herpes simplex* family. The two most common are *herpes simplex type 1* (HSV-1) and *herpes simplex type 2* (HSV-2). These viruses look identical under the microscope, and either type can infect the mouth or genitals. Most commonly, however, HSV-1 occurs above the waist, and HSV-2 below.

While genital herpes can cause symptoms in a variety of sites below the waist, the term is used to denote all HSV infection that is latent in the nerve root at the base of the spine where the virus hides. About two-thirds of people who are infected don't know they have genital herpes, either because they have no symptoms or because their symptoms are so mild they go unnoticed.

Symptoms of the first infection usually appear one to twenty-six days after exposure and last two to three weeks. Symptoms in the genital area include an itching or burning sensation, discharge, and blisters or painful open sores. They are sometimes accompanied by flu-like symptoms such as swollen glands and fever. After the first infection, the virus hides only to reactivate and cause new outbreaks of sores at a later time.

The frequency and severity of these recurrent outbreaks vary. If you suspect you may have herpes, write down your specific symptoms in your health journal and be sure to record the date and the severity of the symptoms. (For a reminder of how to set up a health journal, see Day 7). The next time you visit a doctor, bring your health journal so you won't forget important details.

What does herpes look like?

Symptoms of herpes may or may not be obvious. The herpes virus starts to multiply when it gets into skin cells. The skin becomes red and sensitive. Then one or more blisters will appear. First the blisters open, then they heal as new skin tissue forms over them. During a first outbreak, the area is usually painful. At first you may feel a tingling or itching sensation in the area of your body where a sore is about to appear. You might feel like you're getting the flu—swollen glands, headache, muscle aches, and fever are all common symptoms.

Tiny sores will develop in the spot on your body where the initial infection occurred. These sores are very painful during the initial attack. Once formed, the sore:

- oozes a clear watery liquid
- develops scabs
- heals
- then disappears

Active virus may be present on the skin from the first warning signals (called the **prodrome**) until the sore completely disappears. After the initial outbreak, the severity of symptoms usually decreases with each subsequent outbreak.

What are the symptoms of genital herpes?

Signs and symptoms of genital herpes vary greatly from one episode to the next, and from one person to the next. Breaks or irregularities in the skin (lesions) are often found in recurrent episodes. Some people will notice small sores, and others will have blister-like lesions that eventually crust over. In recurrent outbreaks, however, the healing process usually takes less than half the time than during a first outbreak.

Many people have very subtle forms of recurrent herpes that can heal in a matter of days. These subtle forms of herpes are sometimes mistaken for insect bites, abrasions, yeast, jock itch, hemorrhoids, and other skin conditions. Genital herpes sores are found on the penis or can sometimes also infect the urethra, causing a burning sensation when you urinate. Herpes also can be found on the outside of the vagina. It can also appear near the anus or on the thigh or buttocks—anywhere near the genital area.

What are the symptoms of oral herpes?

Red or white sores or blisters form on the lips, tongue, gums, or roof of the mouth. Herpes labialis (bumpy red sores on the lips) are the most common type of recurrent herpes simplex infections.

How is herpes transmitted?

Among adults, herpes is usually spread through sexual contact, but it can also be transmitted non-sexually. Actually, the highest incidence of the spread of herpes viruses occurs in children through non-sexual contact (usually with oral herpes). Besides genital-to-genital contact, both HSV-1 and HSV-2 can be spread through mouth-to-genital contact or mouth-to-mouth contact. Herpes can be spread through:

○ sexual intercourse (vaginal and anal)
○ mouth-to-mouth sexual contact (kissing)
○ close oral, anal, or genital contact
○ mutual masturbation
○ genital-to-genital contact

A person is considered contagious when he or she has prodromal symptoms (the itching and tingling that come before the outbreak of a herpes sore), active sores, and sores that have begun to heal. Herpes can also be spread by the fingers. If enough active virus touches the skin where it is thin (on the mouth, genitals, or eye areas), or where the skin is broken, cut, or scratched, the virus can enter the body.

Don't forget that herpes can spread from one part of your body to another (called auto-innoculation). If you touch a herpes sore and then touch another area, the virus can infect the new area. Herpes only spreads (from one person to another or from one part of your body to another) when the virus is active, not when it's in remission.

Contrary to popular belief, sores are not always visible or present when the virus is in an active state. Sometimes the virus can spread even when no symptoms are present. This is called **asymptomatic shedding**. Herpes is often transmitted by people who are not aware that they're infected, or by people who simply don't recognize that their herpes infection is in an active phase.

Herpes is spread by direct skin-to-skin contact. For example, if you have a cold sore and you kiss someone, you can transfer the virus from your mouth to theirs. And if you have a cold sore and put your mouth on another person's genitals, you can give that person genital herpes.

Genital herpes and HIV are a bad mix

The CDC recently stated that "HSV infection may adversely affect the progression of immunodeficiency in HIV-infected persons." The CDC notes that people with HIV and HSV are generally more HSV-contagious than people who don't have HIV.

While specific studies in HIV and HSV co-infection have yet to be completed, the CDC suggests there may be a future role for anti-HSV treatment in preventing the spread of HIV, HSV, or to treat with both viruses.

During the 1990s, acyclovir (Zovirax), a drug used to treat herpes, proved to have some benefits in people with HIV. Researchers theorized that when these herpes-related infections happened in people with HIV, they stimulated the activity of the underlying HIV. Researchers also thought that acyclovir might have a direct role in the treatment of HIV because an early HIV study found people taking acyclovir had a 40 percent longer survival, compared to those that did not take the drug. They thought acyclovir might improve the body's response to HIV drugs, but further studies to test this theory failed to show this.

Today, anti-herpes drugs make the most sense when used to fight herpes-related infections in people with HIV. According to Dr. Timothy Schacker, associate director of the Division of Infectious Diseases at the University of Minnesota, who has been studying the herpes-HIV link for more than a decade, "If you are HIV-infected and have herpes, your herpes would recur far more often than if you were not HIV-infected. The insidious thing is that it doesn't cause major disease. But when your herpes reactivates, your HIV replicates with greater efficiency and you have a faster progression of your HIV."

Testing for HSV is a good idea

If you have HIV, it's a good idea to be checked for genital herpes. This includes a new blood test called a "type-specific serological test." Your doctor may not know about the important relationship between HIV and HSV, so you may have to education him or her about this. The blood test for HSV is usually accurate, although false-negative results may occur in some situations. The HSV test is not yet a routine test, so you'll need to ask specifically about one of the following:

○ POCkit HSV-2 (manufactured by Diagnology)
○ HerpeSelect-1 ELISA IgG or HerpeSelect-2 ELISA IgG (manufactured by Focus Technology)
○ HerpeSelect 1 and 2 Immunoblot IgG (manufactured by Focus Technology).

What are the treatments for herpes?

Acyclovir (Zovirax): The use of acyclovir against herpes is well documented. Like other antiviral drugs, acyclovir does not rid the body of the virus, but merely acts to reduce its severity or slow its growth. Still, as antiviral drugs go, acyclovir has been shown to be very safe and has a good record of effectiveness against herpes and other similar conditions.

Valacyclovir (Valtrex): Valacyclovir is effective in suppressing genital herpes outbreaks among people with HIV. One recent study showed that after six months, the proportion of patients who did not have an outbreak was 80 percent in those taking the drug, compared to only 38 percent of those receiving a placebo. Another study showed that the drug lengthened the time between recurrences—for both oral and genital herpes. But the researchers noted that the drug had no impact on HIV viral load.

Famciclovir (Famvir): According to the drug's manufacturer, famciclovir is effective in suppressing genital herpes outbreaks in people with HIV. The company touted one study that found the drug to be about as effective as valacyclovir, and another showed that the drug was superior to acyclovir. However, in June 2000, the drug's manufacturer was warned by government officials for making "misleading safety and efficacy claims, and unsupported superiority claims regarding Famvir."

Topical creams: Topical creams that contain antiviral drug offer little benefit and generally are not recommend. Isolated reports have surfaced indicating success with about topical 5-percent imiquimod cream (Aldara), but research has yet to be completed.

You have choices about treating herpes

With all drugs used to treat herpes, patients can choose between two kinds of treatment. This first is *episodic therapy,* which means taking a drug during an outbreak to speed healing. Another option is *suppressive therapy,* which means taking a drug every day to keep herpes in check, so that it's less likely to flare up and cause symptoms. Suppressive therapy may reduce the number of outbreaks for most people, and may prevent outbreaks altogether for some. It can also greatly reduce asymptomatic shedding (the recurrence of virus on the skin).

Genital warts are caused by a virus

Warts don't come from toads, they come from viruses. The viruses to blame come from a large family called **human papillomavirus (HPV)**. There are about one hundred different members of this family, or strains, of HPV. Some strains of HPV cause warts on the hands (palmar warts) and feet (plantar warts). Other strains of HPV prefer a more tropical environment, such as the warmer and wetter skin in and around your genitals.

Because some strains of HPV reside amid your genitals, they're easily spread from person to person through sexual contact, although this is not always the case. (Of course, you may have had sex with someone who looked like a toad, but that's another story!). When HPV gets into the skin near or on your genitals, it is considered a sexually transmitted disease. HPV can infect the skin of the penis, vulva, labia, or anus, or the tissues covering the vagina and cervix, or anywhere near the genital area. HPV is transmitted in basically the same ways as herpes.

Some strains of HPV are worse than others. Some are considered "high-risk" types and may cause abnormal Pap smears and cancer of the cervix, anus, and penis. Others are "low-risk" and they may cause mild Pap smear abnormalities and genital warts. Genital warts are single or multiple growths or bumps that appear in the genital area, and sometimes form a cauliflower-like shape.

HPV is common among people with HIV

It's estimated that 15 percent of Americans between the ages of 15 to 49 have HPV and rates among men are thought to be similar to those in women. One study of women who were at risk for HIV found that 26 percent of HIV-negative women were infected with HPV, but 70 percent of HIV-positive women had HPV.

Another study of homosexual men found that 60 percent of HIV-negative men had HPV, but almost all HIV-positive individuals had HPV. In other words, if you have HIV there's a good chance you also have HPV. Unfortunately, the two viruses are often travel buddies.

As if growths on the skin aren't bad enough, HPV can also cause your skin to change over time in ways that make it more susceptible to cancer. These skin changes are called **dysplasia**, which is likely to turn into cancer over time. One study suggested that from 20 to 40 percent of people with HIV are likely to be diagnosed with cancer (don't get freaked here because there are things you can do to improve your odds). Cervical cancer caused by HPV is seen far more often in women with lower T-cells. In fact, cervical cancer is considered an AIDS-defining illness.

For both women and men with HIV, the overall risks of anal cancer are significantly higher because of HPV. Research has shown that the risk for anal cancer in men with HIV doubles from 15 to 30 percent as their T-cell count declines. Some researchers have speculated that because people with HIV are living longer due to successful HIV treatment, there may be a significant increase in the incidence of anal cancer.

The good news is that HIV treatment helps to reduce HPV progression, and may reduce the risk of dysplasia or cancer. One study of women on HIV treatment showed they were 1.4 times more likely to experience regression of HPV, while those not on HIV treatments were more likely to have HPV progression. Researchers noted that lowering HIV load and restoring the immune system might retard the progression of cancers due to HPV.

HPV is difficult to see

HPV itself does not cause signs or symptoms, and having HPV does not mean that genital warts will develop. Sometimes, however, HPV does cause warts in or near the genital area that can be felt with a finger or may be visible. Genital warts range from cauliflower-like growths that are easily spotted to smooth bumps. They also may be flat, almost invisible growths. Some warts are hard and rough, others soft and fleshy. They're painless, but may bleed easily or itch.

Common sites in women are on the labia minor, or around the vaginal opening. In men, warts may appear on the head or shaft of the penis. In both men and women, warts can appear in or around the anus. Dysplasia and cancer do not usually cause obvious symptoms.

HPV transmitted by skin-to-skin contact

Genital HPV is only transmitted through skin-to-skin contact. Infected skin of one person rubs against the skin of the other person and transfers the virus. Most HPV is transmitted during vaginal or anal sex, but on rare occasions HPV may be transmitted by mouth-genital sex. Condoms are not as effective at preventing HPV as they are for preventing other STDs, but they can reduce your chances of getting or giving this virus. Condoms don't prevent all skin-to-skin contact during sex. Transmission of HPV is possible when there are no visible signs. Infants born to infected mothers may become infected. HPV can be spread through:

- O sexual intercourse (vaginal and anal)
- O mouth-to-genital contact
- O close oral, anal, or genital contact
- O mutual masturbation
- O genital-to-genital contact

Don't forget that HPV can be spread from one part of your body to another (called auto-innoculation) by touching, scratching, or shaving areas with warts.

Being aggressive about treatment for HPV will pay off

There are no treatments for HPV itself, but there are successful treatments for the warts caused by HPV. Visible warts should be removed—and sooner is always better. Untreated, the warts are very likely to grow in size or multiply in number. It's possible they may go away on their own, but if you have HIV, that's probably not likely. The research to date suggests that removal of visible warts reduces, but does not eliminate, the chances of your spreading them to someone else.

There are many ways to treat genital warts, and there is no definite evidence to say that any one method is superior. Keeping your T-cells as high as possible, quitting smoking (research has documented this), and finding a healthcare professional with experience in treating HPV-related warts are probably your best bets. Warts often come back after treatment, so you'll need to be committed to having them treated several times. Don't be discouraged if they come back.

Treatment for genital warts may include one—or a combination—of the following:

- O podofilox 5% solution or gel
- O imiquimod 5% cream (Aldara)
- O cryotherapy (freezing of the warts)
- O podophyllin resin
- O trichloroacetic acid or bichloroacetic acid
- O surgical removal

○ laser surgery
○ interferon

Pap smears can predict trouble— for women and men

Before the invention of the Pap smear, cervical cancer was the number-one killer of women worldwide. Since the Pap smear, cervical cancer in the United States has dropped by 75 percent. In 1993, federal guidelines required doctors to give women with HIV a cervical Pap smear as part of initial and routine care. A healthcare provider can perform a Pap smear, in which cells are scraped from the cervix and then examined under a microscope.

Although there is some controversy about how often women with HIV should receive Pap smears, it is generally recommended that you have them every six months. If a Pap smear is abnormal, it should be repeated in three months. Women with less than 500 T-cells may have false-negative Pap smears, so shorter intervals between tests might be a good idea.

Men and women who have anal sex should also have regular anal Pap smears to check for dysplasia or cancer. The same procedure is performed, except tissue samples are scraped from the inside of the anus. Pap smears for men are less common, so you may need to educate your doctor about this.

If an abnormal Pap-smear result is found, closer examination will be necessary. At this point, magnifying devices are used to look for dysplasia or cancerous patches inside the anus or cervix. If unusual patches are found, a biopsy should be performed to learn more about the abnormal cells.

Depending on the results of the biopsy, the unusual cells may be given a stage number: I, II, or III. The stage of dysplasia depends on the thickness of abnormal cells within the cervical or anal wall. Stage I is considered to be a mild form of dysplasia and generally does not require therapy, but must be monitored closely. Stages II or III are considered to be more advanced forms of dysplasia and are more likely to develop into cancer. Advanced forms of dysplasia require treatment to prevent them from developing into cancer.

IN A SENTENCE:

> *Herpes and HPV are common sexually transmitted diseases and there are effective treatments for both.*

MONTH **3**

Anxiety, Depression, and Suicide

I TESTED positive for HIV in 1987. During the three months since I had gotten my results, I walked out on my job, quit summer school, and spent most of my time drinking and crying.

The initial shock had subsided, but another emotion began to take its place. At the time, I didn't know there was a specific medical name for what I was feeling. I thought I was just nervous, very nervous. The feeling descended on me when I thought about what was happening to me. I started sweating, my heart began to race, and I couldn't seem to breathe.

A few belts of gin made the feeling go away. But after three months, I was running out of money and excuses for avoiding my family. The pressure mounted until I couldn't take it any longer. So one evening, I set out for a local AIDS organization that was holding a public meeting.

At the meeting, I didn't talk to a soul. I sat in the back, afraid, and somehow expected other people to approach me. When they didn't, when I left the meeting room, I felt so scared and alone that I wanted to die. Then it occurred to me: instead of dealing with money, family, and an ugly disease, I would just kill myself.

At a drugstore, I bought some over-the-counter pills and more gin. Back at my apartment, I sat in the dark wondering. Swallowing all those pills was the easy part. The problem was how I felt after they were down. I got really scared in a pathetic kind of way. I curled up on the floor. At least things would be different, if nothing else.

It wasn't until my stomach started convulsing that I completely chickened out and called a friend. He arrived and when we got to the hospital, I was covered in vomit and couldn't stand upright.

In the emergency room, someone shined a light in one of my eyes. I heard something about a stomach pump, and I was restrained in a chair. A voice said a tube was about to go in my nose and down my throat. On first try, it must have gone down wrong, and I started bleeding. On second try, after gagging and gasping for air, the tube went down.

Suicide is not like it is in the movies, where someone takes some pills, has a few drinks, and neatly drifts off to sleep. In reality, it is a messy, painful, degrading, and ultimately expensive way to get attention. While strapped to that chair, what I remember most was that I didn't want to die at all. I just wanted somebody to help me.

Having HIV is easier these days

Back in 1987, having HIV was a different thing. People were hysterical, there were no treatments, and it really was considered a death sentence. For people testing positive today, everything about the disease is so drastically improved that, by all measures, it's truly a chronic, manageable condition. I am proof of that.

However, breakthroughs in medicine and improved social acceptance of the disease don't always change how people feel when they first test positive. Emotions don't always respond to statistics.

You may be facing any number of challenges in your life beyond HIV. Testing positive might feel like the straw that breaks the camel's back. You may feel a loss of control over your life, or a variety of overwhelming fears. These feelings may hit you all at once, or they may come and go, depending on other factors in your life.

On the other hand, you may be coping well. Perhaps you had expected the diagnosis and were aware of the advances in treatment. Maybe you have friends with HIV who are well and happy. If this is the case, you're lucky. However, don't dismiss the subtle emotional impact that HIV can have as you go about your business.

Either way, understanding your feelings—and knowing how you might respond to certain situations down the road—can help in adjusting better and more quickly to the changes in your life during the next year.

Anxiety, depression, and thoughts of suicide are normal for anyone facing a major medical condition, including HIV. The Living section of this chapter explores some of the typical reactions that people might have after testing positive. The Learning section offers some potential actions and treatments for these conditions.

Above all, if you begin to feel overwhelmed by any emotion, or find yourself in a numb or emotionless state, the most important thing you can do is to ask for help.

Anxiety starts with persistent worrying

Anxiety is not easy to define. It is a disturbance of your mood or emotional tone. It can start as a sense of worry, stress, or nervousness about an anticipated event or outcome.

The likelihood of developing anxiety probably involves life experiences, your psychological makeup, and genetic factors. Men tend to experience more anxiety than women; however, it is not entirely clear why.

Mild-to-moderate anxiety is very common. Symptoms may include excessive worrying, agitation, shakiness, irritability, feeling "on edge" or "hyper," muscle tension, difficulty concentrating or falling asleep, and changes in appetite. Certainly, testing positive for HIV is a major life event and mild-to-moderate anxiety can be expected with varying degrees and at different times.

More pronounced or persistent anxiety can be classified as a medical condition called an anxiety disorder. The lifetime prevalence of anxiety disorders in the United States is between 10 and 15 percent. Reports have confirmed that increased anxiety—often lasting up to several months—are common in the course of living with HIV. However, specific anxiety disorders appear to be no more common in people with HIV than in the general population. Symptoms of some anxiety disorders include:

○ **Generalized Anxiety Disorder.** Medically speaking, generalized anxiety disorder is when you persistently have vague feelings that something bad is going to happen. Excessive or unrealistic worries are often so persistent that you cannot make them go away, or you have difficulty concentrating on daily tasks.

○ **Panic Disorder.** Panic disorder is when you feel unexpected and repeated episodes of intense fear accompanied by physical symptoms such as your heart beginning to race, chest pains, shortness of breath, dizziness, nausea, numbness, trembling, abdominal distress, and a fear of going crazy or dying. The attack usually hits abruptly, building in intensity within ten to fifteen minutes. You may feel you want to flee from the location where the "panic attack" started. Attacks usually last no more than thirty minutes.

○ **Post-Traumatic Stress Disorder.** Post-traumatic stress disorder usually happens after a terrifying event, causing repeated frightening thoughts and memories. Ordinary events can trigger flashbacks or intrusive images. People may become easily irritated or have violent outbursts. One recent study of ethnically diverse women found up to 42 percent of women who sought treatment for HIV met the criteria for this disorder.

It's normal to worry when you have HIV

If you just found out you have HIV, who could blame you for being worried? But you're not alone in your concerns. The psychological impact of HIV has been fairly well studied by researchers and mental health professionals who have found many common themes. Among them are:

○ **Fear of the unknown.** If you don't know much about HIV, you might believe you won't live much longer.

○ **The unpredictable nature of HIV.** When your blood tests are good, you may feel elated, but when they're down, you may feel worry and anxiety.

○ **Fear of stigmatization.** Gay men, intravenous drug users, and sex trade workers are already stigmatized by society. You might feel HIV will bring about more labeling, rejection, isolation, or discrimination.

○ **Being a hypochondriac.** You might become obsessed with minor illnesses or fluctuations in your body. You might spend too much time checking your lymph nodes, your skin, or your mouth.

○ **Pressure to maintain a positive attitude.** You might feel as if you should be optimistic all the time. The pressure might be aggravated by faulty reports that self-affirmation, laughter, and positive thinking can control the disease.

Depression can slowly creep into your life

I wish I could report that things got better after my suicide attempt, that I got the help I actually needed, and that it was smooth sailing afterward. But it's rare when big problems in life get fixed in simple ways.

A few months passed. I managed to hold down a job, which helped with finances and kept my mind occupied. I drank less, probably because I conned different doctors into prescribing me tranquilizers. With each doctor, I recited the same sob story about "fear of dying with AIDS." Hence, I maintained a steady supply of sedatives and sleeping pills.

I thought I was coping fairly well with anxiety, which seemed to ease. However, what seemed to take its place was, well, a lack of emotions, a numbness and apathy. This lack of concern was not just about my health situation, but about life in general. On a good day, my moods were neutral. Slowly and subtly over time, I lost the desire to have fun. Fun was lowering the shades, downing a few tranquilizers, eating Haagen-Daz, and watching Bugs Bunny reruns.

I slept a lot. In fact, I disliked waking. Whenever I woke up, I had a few good moments until I was hit with the reality of my situation. My running joke was that sleeping was the only way to be alive and unconscious at the same time. Soon, I gained weight, felt worse, and the vicious cycle was in motion.

Depression is not sadness and it is not a character flaw

Depression is more than feeling sad, although people often use the term depression to describe sadness. Sadness or the "blues" are actually short-lived, unhappy feelings that occur in response to a particular event. They generally fade with time, or as the event resolves or improves.

As with anxiety, true depression is a chronic medical condition. It's a potentially severe, brain chemical imbalance that interferes with normal functioning—and 15 percent of the time, it resolves by suicide.

Unlike anxiety, depression is about twice as common in women as in men. About one in ten Americans experiences chronic depression, while the rates for people with HIV are estimated at about one in three, making it the most common psychiatric disorder among this group. While just the thought of having HIV may seem depressing, the true underlying reasons may be that depression-prone people are more likely to get HIV in the first

Are You Depressed?

DOCTORS USE specific guidelines to determine if someone is clinically depressed. If you have five of the following nine symptoms every day for at least two weeks, you're likely to have major depression. You should discuss these symptoms with your healthcare provider.

1. **Depressed mood**

   This isn't just rainy days or Mondays. This is deep, unrelenting sadness that may even "color" the way you see normal things in your life.

2. **Diminished interest or pleasures**

   When I was depressed, I didn't return phone calls, I didn't make plans with other people, I didn't exercise, and I really didn't care.

3. **Weight changes**

   Most people lose weight, I gained weight.

4. **Sleeping too much or too little**

   Persistent changes in your normal sleep patterns may signal depression. If I start sleeping more than my normal eight hours, I know something is wrong.

5. **Restlessness or inactivity**

   After waking, I would lie around in my robe for hours, smoking cigarettes, drinking coffee, and never get much accomplished. Then, I was late to work.

6. **Fatigue or loss of energy**

   This is a constant heaviness, particularly in the arms and legs. Some people feel as if they're carrying around a cinder block. I dreaded the idea of climbing stairs, especially with groceries.

7. **Feelings of worthlessness or guilt**

   Classic symptoms, these feelings may become exaggerated far beyond what people without depression would feel in the same circumstances. I often obsessed about the idea of disappointing my parents.

8. **Inability to think clearly**

   Most people are a little slow or groggy when they first wake up from sleep. Depressed people may feel as they can't shake off this grogginess all day long.

9. **Suicidal thoughts**

   Testing positive for HIV makes people think about mortality. Dying or funeral fantasies are human and normal. But when these thoughts persist over time or grow in seriousness, that's not normal.

place. Some research even suggests that HIV itself may play a role in clinical depression. Without question, depression manifests in other chronic viral conditions such as hepatitis B or hepatitis C.

An interesting study recently found that, although death rates among women with HIV have decreased in the United States since the introduction of new HIV treatments, the proportion of deaths caused by non-AIDS-related conditions has remained steady at about 20 percent. Researchers reported that the majority of non-AIDS-related deaths were related to depression and substance abuse. I'm sure there are many parallels here for men as well.

Depression is not a character flaw. It's not laziness or a lack of motivation. It's an abnormally low level of a brain chemical called **serotonin**, the brain chemical that helps humans cope with stresses from the outside world. Low levels of serotonin are linked to all kinds of unhealthy behavior, such as overeating, aggression, alcoholism, drug addiction, and compulsive behaviors.

If you have five of the symptoms listed on page 121, you're clinically depressed. The Learning section will discuss some options for you. However, if you have four of these symptoms, that doesn't mean you're fine. Depression can wax and wane, come and go. It's a good idea to write down any symptoms in your health journal and track them over time. This way, you can track any symptoms of depression over time and then discuss them in detail with your doctor. In fact, tracking the details of depression with a health journal may even help you and your doctor decide your next steps.

Many people don't acknowledge depression

Many people see depression as a sign of weakness, so they don't acknowledge the depth of their condition. That's one way to deal with the situation. But research shows that depression is associated with higher rates of mortality in people with HIV. The cause and effect of an HIV diagnosis and depression is not always clear. What's clear is that relief is out there—if that's what you want. The Learning section of this chapter is devoted to ways to deal with depression as well as anxiety.

Thinking about suicide is normal, planning it is not

Researchers in France recently discovered that among HIV-positive people who had a good response from HIV treatment, one in ten committed suicide. These were people with high T-cells and low viral loads.

In general, people don't think about suicide too often. Most people are familiar with the term "physician-assisted suicide," where a trained doctor provides a patient the tools needed to commit suicide. In these cases, a terminally ill patient then takes action to end his or her own life, usually to alleviate intense physical pain that comes with certain conditions or diseases.

For people with end-stage AIDS, physician-assisted suicide is a consideration. For people who are testing positive now, occasional suicidal fantasies may be a way to cope, or a rare thought now and then. My favorite suicide fantasy is being hit by a bus. People always told me that "everyone is going to die someday; I could get hit by a bus tomorrow." I should be so lucky.

Don't worry about suicidal thoughts until you start working out the details of your plan. If you find yourself planning for something, you are not in your best frame of mind. Think about it, if the better option is to kill yourself, you are beyond miserable. And if you feel that bad, let someone help you. Talk to someone.

You might not believe it now, but relief is possible. It might come in the form of talking with another person, taking medicine, or spiritual belief. But if you're not receptive to the idea that things can get better, you'll have a harder time finding relief.

Suicide Hotline

FOR CRISIS CALLS: (800) 784-2433

IN A SENTENCE:

> *Anxiety, depression, and fleeting thoughts of suicide are common and normal, but planning suicide is a serious sign that you might need help.*

learning

Fixing the Funk: Treating Anxiety and Depression

ANXIETY AND depression are the most common reasons that people with HIV seek assistance with mental health. The two conditions are different, but related. They can occur independently of each other at different times, or together at once. You can have depression with occasional periods of anxiety. On the other hand, you could be experiencing anxiety with occasional bouts of depression. Some treatments help both depression and anxiety at the same time.

If you suspect that depression or anxiety may be an issue for you, chances are that you will do one of the following:

○ do nothing and hope the conditions resolve
○ try behavior modification techniques such as regular exercise, yoga, or meditation
○ explore herbal supplements (not recommended if you're taking any other medications)
○ pursue psychotherapy (talking with a trained mental health professional)
○ try prescription medications
○ combine several of these approaches

Doing nothing is one option

Doing nothing for anxiety or depression is certainly an option that many people choose. Sure, you can pull the sheets over your head and hope for the best. Sometimes, clinical depression can lift on its own in six to twelve months. Sometimes, anxiety lessens with time as you become adjusted to living with HIV. But if these conditions turn severe or persist for extended periods of time, doing nothing will make things worse. Major depression in people with HIV is associated with decreased survival, increased hospital stays, and impaired quality of life. And 15 percent of depressed people take their own lives.

Exercise, yoga, or meditation can help

Exercise, yoga, and meditation might help—and can't hurt—in combating depression and anxiety. Research has shown exercise can have a positive impact on depression. You should already know this: Moving your body is good for your health. It's clearly documented that regular exercise improves depression. But you don't need science to tell you that exercise improves your mood. Some people swear by yoga as a way to battle anxiety. They say that by focusing on the stretching and attaining the postures, you can tune out persistent or negative thoughts. Meditation may work in a similar way.

Herbal supplements may help with some conditions

Herbal supplements to treat anxiety and depression are controversial. Still, two-thirds of people with HIV use some form of alternative medicine. Many people don't tell their doctor that they are experimenting with herbs. If you're not currently taking HIV treatment or other medications, there's much less potential harm from herbal supplements interacting with your drugs. In this case, testing out a few herbs is one way to see if they work for you. ***Here are some supplements that some people have used:***

St. John's Wort

St. John's Wort (*Hypericum performatum*) is a popular herbal supplement used to treat mild to moderate depression. Some scientific studies have shown this plant-based herb is effective, although a more recent study casts doubt on previous findings. It is not effective for more serious or chronic depression. Research has shown that there are serious and potentially harmful interactions with many conventional drugs, notably some forms of HIV treatments. If you're not taking HIV treatment or other medications, experimenting with this supplement has fewer risks.

KAVA

Kava (*Piper methysticum*) is a plant that has become popular for its reported ability to relieve stress, anxiety, tension, and sleeplessness. It is often used as an ingredient in dietary supplements and herbal teas. However, such products have been associated with serious liver-related injuries, including hepatitis, cirrhosis, and liver failure. The US Food and Drug Administration (FDA) has issued a warning to consumers about the potential risks, especially for people who may have pre-existing liver problems.

Psychotherapy (talk therapy) and support groups can keep you sane

Talking with other people has kept me from losing my marbles during my fifteen years of having HIV. Let me be clear about this, what's kept me sane over the years has been talking with other people in a structured and therapeutic environment. By structured and therapeutic, I mean a setting with some ground rules and a sense of purpose. Chatting with friends or family about your concerns does not always fall into this category (and, in fact, is sometimes counterproductive).

Talk therapy can take place in a group setting or one on one. Group settings can range from highly structured to very informal. For example, many AIDS organizations offer structured group therapy for people with HIV. The groups are usually limited in number, anywhere from five to twelve individuals per group. The groups usually meet once a week over the course of eight to twelve weeks. They are usually headed by a trained professional who helps guide the conversation and enforces ground rules.

For me, group therapy was a lifesaver. At first I felt awkward about sharing my feelings with strangers. As I learned more about the others in the group, I eventually got more comfortable. I felt less alone with my problems. In fact, other people in the group often described exactly what I was going through. Sometimes, they offered solutions that hadn't occurred to me. I didn't like everyone in the group—some I even despised. At times, group therapy seemed corny, melodramatic, and even depressing. Still, the groups eased my anxiety and fear about HIV.

Finding a therapist can make you crazy

One-on-one talk therapy, also called **psychotherapy** or counseling, is a whole different thing. When you seek out mental healthcare, you'll find a lot of confusing choices. Some of those choices may be limited by what you can afford, what your insurance covers, or what kind of access you have to health organizations. There's a list of resources on page 274 to help you get started.

Mental health professionals who offer one-on-one talk therapy are often called "therapists" but this is an umbrella term that refers to a broad range of services. There are many types of licensed and unlicensed mental health professionals. They differ in educational backgrounds, training, state licensing, philosophy, and technique.

In the same way that you should interview potential new doctors, you should also interview therapists about their experience and training. You'll do best if you find someone with whom you share some values or experiences. The next step is figuring out if the mental health professional has experience with the type of problems you're having. Experience with HIV is a good idea. Some therapists offer a free initial consultation by phone or in person to help assess if they're right for you.

Here's a brief overview of the types of mental health professionals, their education, licenses, and certifications:

○ **Psychiatrists** are medical doctors, and can prescribe medication. Very few psychiatrists provide psychotherapy, but usually refer you to a psychotherapist. If you need medication, you will usually have to see a psychiatrist.

○ **Psychologists** usually have a doctorate degree and have completed an internship under supervision.

○ **Counselors** usually have a master's degree in counseling and have completed an internship under supervision, but not always. Counselors usually specialize in specific areas such as substance abuse, anxiety, or short-term crises.

○ **Clinical social workers** typically have a master's degree in social work and have completed a supervised internship.

ACADEMIC DEGREES:
M.A.—Master of Arts
M.S.—Master of Science

M.S.W.—Master of Social Work
Ph.D.—Doctor of Philosophy
Ed.D.—Doctor of Education
Psy.D.—Doctor of Psychology
M.Ed –Master of Educational Psychology
M.D.—Doctor of Medicine

LICENSES AND CERTIFICATIONS:
C.A.C.—Certified Addictions Counselor
C.S.W.—Certified Social Worker
C.S.W.—Clinical Social Worker
L.L.P.—Limited License Psychologist
L.P.—Licensed Psychologist
L.P.C.—Licensed Professional Counselor
L.M.F.T.—Licensed Marriage and Family Therapist
S.W.—Social Worker
P.C.C. or L.P.C.C.—Professional Clinical Counselors
C.P.C.—Certified Professional Counselor

The therapist-patient relationship may reflect other relationships

The weird thing about therapy is that the relationship between you and your therapist often reflects the relationships you have with other people in your life. For example, you might find a therapist with whom you're initially comfortable. But with time, you might start avoiding certain topics or missing appointments. You may even think you have good reasons for avoiding issues or missing sessions. What might be happening, however, is that you're uncomfortable with intimate relationships or afraid of being yourself. It may turn out that you're having the same problems with other people in your life.

On the other hand, you might get hooked up with a therapist who genuinely doesn't share your values or experiences. You might disagree about philosophical, social, cultural, or sexual issues. You are the only person who can determine if the therapist isn't right for you. I've certainly encountered therapists who've said or done things that disturbed me to the core. One therapist fell asleep on me in the middle of my session. Another said that I wasn't born "normal." In those cases, I knew the particular therapists weren't right for me.

At other points in my life, I had a great therapist who pushed me emotionally. This, too, was difficult—but in a good way. Often, I became angry at my therapist. Sometimes I resented the weekly appointment. Once, I failed to show up at all—for several weeks. But somehow I knew it wasn't the therapist; it was me being stubborn. When I stuck out, when I continued to talk despite feeling uncomfortable, the payoff was worth the pain: I learned entirely new ways of seeing myself and the world around me.

Prescription drugs can help with mood disorders

Today's drugs for depression and anxiety are not your mother's drugs for depression and anxiety. In terms of depression, drug therapy has come a long way. The first generation of antidepressants was introduced in the 1950s. This class of drugs was dubbed **tricyclics** for their three-ringed molecular structure.

Although the trycyclics provide relief from depression, they were biochemically clumsy and produced several side effects. The class of drugs includes

- amitriptypline (Elavil)
- nortriptyline (Pamelor)
- desipramine (Norpramin)

Not much later came another class of drugs called **monoamine oxidase inhibitors (MAOIs)**. Monoamine oxidase is an enzyme inside some nerves. Inhibition of this enzyme allows more norepinephrin, dopamine, and serotonin to be produced. The three neurotransmitters are linked to moods and sleep. Decreased levels are associated with depressed moods. Common MAOIs include

- phenelzine (Nardil)
- tranylcypromine (Parnate)

The biggest problem with both types of these early antidepressants is their potential for serious side effects. MAOIs interact with certain foods to cause a sudden rise in blood pressure. Also, MAOIs sometimes produced tremors, insomnia, weight gain, and liver toxicity. Tricyclics can cause reduced mental acuity, drowsiness, dry mouth, blurred vision, weight gain, and sexual dysfunction.

Prozac-like drugs are very effective in reducing depression

By the late 1980s, a third generation of antidepressants became available to consumers. The new drugs, called selective serotonin reuptake inhibitors (SSRIs), have profound advantages over MAOIs and trycyclics. SSRIs are easier to tolerate because of their relative lack of unpleasant side effects, and they relieve depression about as effectively as the older medications. This new generation of antidepressants includes

- ○ fluoxetine (Prozac)
- ○ paroxetine (Paxil)
- ○ sertraline (Zoloft)
- ○ fluvoxamine (Luvox)
- ○ nefazadone (Serzone)

SSRIs are the most prescribed class of antidepressants. SSRIs have fewer interactions with other medications and are not associated with the weight gain common in people taking tricyclics. Also, SSRIs have a wide margin of safety in overdose and do not appear to be associated with withdrawal symptoms.

A relative of the SSRI family is a group of antidepressants called **partial serotonin reuptake inhibitors**. The mechanism of action for these related drugs is slightly different from standard SSRIs. In some cases, partial serotonin reuptake inhibitors may produce different side effects. These drugs include

- ○ venlafaxine (Effexor)
- ○ buspropian (Wellbutrin)

Anti-anxiety drugs can help you deal with panic

Symptoms of anxiety are relatively easy to treat with prescription drugs. They are widely prescribed—and widely abused as well. If you're prone to substance abuse or are in recovery from drugs or alcohol, you should be careful about your intake of certain drugs used to treat anxiety. Certain classes of drugs may trigger a relapse or complicate the situation. In general, medications to treat anxiety are quite safe, have minimal side effects, and carry little danger of overdosing.

Benzodiazepines are the largest class of drugs used to treat anxiety. They work best if used for short periods of time to manage severe or occasional anxiety. The entire class of drugs may cause some "clouding" of the mind and "slowing" of motor skills. Some benzodiazepines stay in your body longer than others. Discuss with your doctor the risk and benefits of taking benzodiazepines, especially if you have addiction tendencies. The class of drugs includes

- ❍ lorazepam (Ativan and others)
- ❍ alprazolam (Xanax)
- ❍ clonazepam (Klonopin)
- ❍ temazepam (Restoril)

Buspirone (BuSpar) is an alternative to the benzodiazepines. It is not sedating, has few if any mental side effects, and does not create dependency or addiction. Its major drawback is the long period before it takes effect, up to four weeks.

If you decide to pursue medication for anxiety or depression, it's a good idea to track any symptoms or any side effects from medication in your health journal. If, down the road, you and your doctor decide to switch or add medications, the details in your health journal can be especially useful.

IN A SENTENCE:

Anxiety and depression occur among people with HIV and there are several options for treating these conditions.

MONTH **4**

living

Substance Abuse

THIS IS a true story: A while ago, a friend of mine asked his doctor what his chances were of dying from AIDS.

"Honestly?" the doctor asked.

"Honestly," said my friend, thinking that his doctor's response was kind of dumb.

"Well, to be perfectly honest," he said, "I think it's more likely you'll die from drunk driving or a drug overdose than you will from AIDS."

My friend was stunned, speechless even, as if he had just been slapped.

"You asked," the doctor said.

To which my friend, the patient, replied "Yeah, well, remind me not to ask that question again."

He left the office a little dazed, but more irritated than anything else. After all, he assumed he didn't drink *that* much. He didn't drink any more than his friends did. And the drug stuff? Well, prescription drugs don't really count as "drugs." He experimented with party drugs only on occasion. Well, there was that period a few months ago when things got a little out of control. . . .

The worlds of substance abuse and HIV are colliding. These days, HIV clinics are becoming substance abuse clinics and HIV doctors are getting plenty of on-the-job training in addiction medicine. A recent study found that nearly 26 percent of people with HIV used illicit drugs—and that doesn't even count marijuana. The research found that more than 12 percent were drug dependent. This coupled with intravenous drug use accounts for about 30 percent of new HIV cases in the United States.

Here's the deal: If you have HIV and you want to live longer, taking mind-altering substances is probably not the path you want to pursue. If you have HIV and you don't want to live as long as possible, hey, continue taking drugs. Knock yourself out. If your goal is to live longer, here are a few reasons why you should worry about putting mind-altering substances into your body:

○ Such substances result in impaired thinking, which puts you at risk for more health problems.
○ They place stress on the body, which is already burdened by HIV.
○ They reduce your chance of success with HIV treatment.

Addiction starts with a genetic tendency

Genes are like the instruction manual for a human body. Your genes control your height, skin color, hair, and most everything else. Genes are responsible for how your brain works at birth, almost like the factory settings for a new TV. Of course, once you start using your brain and start interacting with your environment, the channels get changed. Both your genes and your environment create the person you are today.

Some genes control how your brain responds to chemicals, such as the ones found in tobacco and alcohol. If you have certain genes, drinking or smoking probably feels great. If you don't have these genes, drinking or smoking probably feels good—but not great. It's the same story for eating, sex, gambling, shopping, or anything else related to pleasure.

If your genes predispose you to substance abuse, it's not a done deal. You and your environment get votes on the issue. You may be predisposed to alcoholism, but because you choose not to drink, you may not be an alcoholic. Maybe you're built to love heroin, but you just haven't tried it.

First-time drug use is a choice

So what turns occasional substance use into substance abuse? "The brain," says Alan Leshner, director of the National Institute on Drug Abuse (NIDA) at the National Institutes of Health. Just as people don't start out intending to get lung cancer when they smoke, or to get clogged arteries when they eat fatty foods, people don't intend to become drug addicts when they first use drugs.

"Initial drug use is a voluntary and therefore a preventable behavior," says Leshner. "However, drug addiction is a disease, a treatable disease that's expressed as a compulsive behavior." According to Leshner, drug addiction is the result of biochemical processes.

While all illicit drugs have different effects on the brain, they also have a common bond: They trigger the release of dopamine, a brain chemical that is directly involved in the experience of pleasure. Feeling good about a job well done, getting pleasure from family or social interactions, feeling content, or feeling that one's life is meaningful, all rely on dopamine. Drug addicts are addicted specifically to the meaningful dopamine spikes that drugs produce in the brain.

"While we haven't yet pinpointed precisely all the triggers for the changes in the brain's structure and function, a vast body of hard evidence shows that it is virtually inevitable that prolonged drug use will lead to addiction," said Leshner. "From this, we can soundly conclude that drug addiction is a brain disease."

People use drugs for two reasons

People use drugs to feel good (sensation-seeking) or to feel better (self-medicating). "The sensation seekers are looking for a novel or exciting experience," says Leshner. "The self-medicating types are attempting to escape life conditions, such as poverty or untreated mental disorders, using drugs as if they were treating anxiety or depression."

Whatever the initial reason for using drugs, the vast majority of people addicted to drugs cannot stop. "The reason for this is that prolonged drug use changes the brain in fundamental and long-lasting ways," say Leshner. "In some sense, the brain is actually rewired as a function of drug use.

Leshner notes that there is something unique about administering drugs to yourself. For example, when doctors give morphine for pain, patients do not become addicted. In this case, patients may develop physical dependence on morphine, but the compulsion to abuse morphine does not become manifest—and compulsion is the essence of addiction.

The notion that drug addiction is a character flaw—that those addicted to drugs are just too weak to quit on their own—"flies in the face of scientific evidence," says Leshner. Therefore, the notion of addiction-as-failure-of-character should be discarded. Instead, he suggests focusing on improving drug-treatment systems, similar to those for treating other chronic relapsing conditions like asthma or hypertension.

Smoking cigarettes will shorten your life

If you have HIV, you're probably already a smoker. Like it or not, studies have shown that the type of people who smoke are the type of people who get HIV. In case you've been living under a rock, smoking causes a number of serious illnesses, from heart disease to cancer. Clearly, quitting smoking is a better choice for improved health. Tobacco and HIV—each on their own—can shorten your life. Together, they're like the perfect storm.

If you have HIV and you smoke, you're more likely to develop the "garden variety" problems associated with smoking. One recent study found that HIV-positive smokers were nearly eight times more likely to develop emphysema than smokers without the virus.

Another study published in 2003 found the incidence of lung cancer has increased in HIV-positive patients treated at the U.K.'s largest HIV clinic since the introduction of the new HIV treatments in 1996. The investigators concluded that since the new treatments, the incidence of HIV-related lung cancer has probably increased because people with HIV are living longer.

People with HIV like to drink

Alcohol dependence rates for both men and women with HIV substantially exceed those in the general population. Some say that between 30 and 70 percent of people with HIV are dependent on alcohol. Men are especially at risk. Sure, booze is legal, but it doesn't mean it's good for your health. Heavy alcohol directly assaults your liver—and after a few years, especially with HIV treatment—the damage to your health can add up.

If you also happen to have chronic hep C or hep B, drinking any alcohol will speed the pace of liver damage. Light-to-moderate use can lead you to behave in ways that may be further damaging to your health. Having HIV doesn't rule out the possibility of a car crash.

If you're considering HIV treatment—or are already taking HIV treatment—you should know that alcohol reduces your chances of success with HIV treatment over the long haul. Why? Alcohol use has a bad effect on

- metabolism of HIV drugs (alcohol changes the way your body absorbs the medicine)

○ adherence (you might choose to drink instead of taking your meds)
○ the balance between the virus and the immune system (to some degree, drinking does have a negative effect on your T-cells and viral load)

"The message to the physician and to the patients is to be aware that this can be very insidious," says Anthony S. Fauci, M.D., director of the National Institute of Allergy and Infectious Diseases. "It would really be a shame, that after all one has been through—finally getting your viral load down to below detectable levels, getting your hepatitis under control, being tested for cervical cancer or anal carcinoma from HPV—after all that, you end up knocking yourself out with chronic liver disease because you're drinking too much. Again, it's part of the whole health picture."

Marijuana is a drug

Some people don't consider marijuana to be a true "drug." Whatever you consider marijuana to be, the real culprit in marijuana is **tetrahydro-cannabinol (THC)**. In the same way that nicotine is the active ingredient in tobacco, THC is the active ingredient in marijuana. THC is responsible for the "high" feeling that your brain learns to love so much.

Is THC addictive? Maybe. According to NIDA, addiction is characterized by "compulsive, at times uncontrollable, drug craving, seeking, and use that persists even in the face of extremely negative consequences." Now, think for a moment and ask yourself this question: Is THC addictive for you?

THC and related chemicals have received attention as a treatment for HIV-related weight loss and nausea. The bottom line is that many people with HIV smoke marijuana. A recent study revealed "no significant immunologic or virologic impact of marijuana" in people with HIV. The researchers did note a decline in testosterone levels, which confirmed findings of several other studies.

Besides the effects on brain chemistry, smoking marijuana carries the same harmful risks associated with burning something—and then sucking it into your lungs. In addition, marijuana is sometimes contaminated with insecticides, pesticides, fungus, and bacteria. Some HIV doctors suggest microwaving marijuana for ten to thirty seconds, especially to kill a nasty fungus called **aspergillosis**.

• • •

Valium and Xanax are benzodiazepines

Who could blame you for not being able to sleep? Or for being nervous? That's precisely why people with HIV tend to have access to benzodiazepines. Doctors often prescribe "benzos" for insomnia and anxiety. Chemically speaking, benzos cling to the central nervous system, causing anything from slight impairment to hypnosis. They're often called "sedatives" or "tranquilizers."

For some, the balance between "medicine" and "drug" is a never-ending tread on a tightrope. Discontinuing prolonged use of high-dose benzodiazepines can lead to serious withdrawal symptoms because all benzos work by slowing the brain's activity. A potential consequence of abuse is that, when you stop, the brain's activity can rebound to the point of causing a seizure. If you're thinking about stopping your benzos, you should seek medical help beforehand.

Benzodiazepines come in a variety of shapes and colors. The most popular way to get the drug is by prescription. The benzodiazepines are a big family and they differ somewhat in side effects, potencies, timing, and the tendency to cause withdrawal. Drugs in the benzodiazepine family include

- alprazolam (Xanax)
- lorazepam (Ativan)
- diazepam (Valium or Valrelease)
- oxazepam (Serax)
- temazepam (Restoril)
- flurazepam (Dalmane)
- triazolam (Halcion).

Cocaine is tough on your heart

Cocaine is a chemical processed from the leaves of the South American shrub *Erythroxylon coca*. A stimulant, cocaine induces a sense of exhilaration in users, mostly by causing dopamine levels to spike.

Crack and cocaine are the same drug. Crack is the street name given to the freebase form of cocaine processed from the powdered cocaine hydrochloride form to a smokable substance.

The term "crack" refers to the crackling sound heard when the mixture is smoked. Crack cocaine is processed with ammonia or baking soda and water, and then heated to remove the hydrochloride. Because crack is smoked, the user experiences a high in seconds.

Chest pain is the most common cocaine-related side effect. That's because cocaine puts stress on your heart. Complications of cocaine abuse also include

- myocarditis
- dilated cardiomyopathy
- myocardial ischemia and infarction
- congestive heart failure
- cardiac arrhythmias

Since 1993, an increasing number of people with HIV have reported heart problems. The heart complications in people with HIV can occur at any stage of HIV and include

- myocarditis
- dilated cardiomyopathy
- pericardial
- endocardial
- rhythm
- vascular abnormalities

One study suggested that among cocaine users, about 17 percent also had HIV. In the United States, up to 6 percent of people with HIV will die from heart problems. The overlap of cocaine abuse and HIV seems obvious, especially as people with HIV live longer.

On the bright side, research is emerging on ways to treat cocaine addiction and its related heart conditions among people with HIV. One recent study examined the role of **angiotensin converting enzyme (ACE) inhibitors**, now commonly used to treat hypertension.

ACE inhibitors have been used in cocaine-abusing populations. They may change the levels of dopamine in the brain, which may help to reduce cocaine abuse. Cocaine abusers who are HIV-positive often have abnormal heart and platelet functions that are potentially reversible with ACE-inhibitors.

Crystal meth is a supercharged amphetamine

A friend describes using crystal meth in this way: "It's evil. You lose all grip. You lose sight of reality until you start losing things, like your car."

The long name for crystal meth is **methamphetamine**. Amphetamine means "powerful stimulant that affects the central nervous system." Crystal meth is the bully of the amphetamine family. The drug is cheap, lasts a long time, and goes by the name of "meth," "speed," "crystal," "crank," or "Tina."

The drug is a white, odorless, bitter-tasting powder that easily dissolves in water or alcohol. Crystal meth was developed early in this century from its parent drug, amphetamine, and was used originally in nasal decongestants and bronchial inhalers.

Amphetamines excite your nervous system, which increases your heart rate and breathing. Your hands may become sweaty as your body heats up, and you lose your appetite. Generally, users feel energetic, alert, talkative, or sexually aroused.

A word of caution

BE VERY cautious if you're taking illicit drugs along with an HIV treatment called **ritonovir**. Ritonovir is often included in various combinations of HIV treatment. Ritonovir has the ability to slow down your liver so it takes longer to eliminate illicit drugs from your blood. This can mean that the dose of illicit drugs in your blood may increase, sometimes by severalfold and sometimes to dangerous levels. If you are taking ritonovir, you might consider experimenting with lower doses of illicit drugs at first to reduce your risks.

Afterward, users feel washed out or depressed. If you've been "tweaking" for several days, lack of sleep or not eating may put a strain on your immune system. The drug seems to be associated with rougher sex, which may lead to bleeding and abrasions. Because a run on crystal meth can strain your immune system, some users get outbreaks of herpes, if they already have herpes. The drug has also been implicated in the spread of hep B and hep C.

Long-term use disrupts the chemical balance within your brain. Researchers have reported that as many as 50 percent of the dopamine-producing cells in the brain can be damaged after prolonged exposure to low levels of crystal meth. Also, serotonin levels are disturbed, which can lead to depression or anxiety.

• • •

Ecstasy is a psychedelic amphetamine

Ecstasy, or **methylenedioxymethamphetamine (MDMA)**, is part hallucinogen and part stimulant. Ecstasy has LSD-like properties, but it's more closely related to amphetamines.

In high doses, Ecstasy can cause a sharp increase in body temperature, leading to muscle breakdown and kidney and heart failure. You might feel muscle tension and start to grind your teeth. You might feel nausea, experience blurred vision, or suffer from rapid eye movement, faintness, and chills or sweating. The drug also destroys serotonin-producing cells in the brain—not a good thing if you're prone to depression or anxiety.

Heroin started as a prescription drug

Heroin deserves a special place in medical history. A derivative of morphine, the drug's real name is **diacetylmorphine**. Heroin is the name that the Bayer Company gave to the drug in 1898. At the time, the drug was a blockbuster like today's Viagra. It took years for the medical profession to figure out the dangers of heroin addiction. Over time, the drug fell out of favor as "medicine" and became popular as a "drug."

Heroin is chemically created from morphine, a naturally occurring substance extracted from the seeds of certain poppy plants. Morphine is a member of a class of drugs also called "opiates" or "narcotics." Other members of this class include hydrocodone (Vicidin) and codeine (Tylenol with Codeine).

- ❍ Heroin is typically sold as a white or brownish powder, or as the black sticky substance called "black tar heroin."
- ❍ It is usually injected, snorted, or smoked.
- ❍ Intravenous injection provides the greatest intensity and most rapid onset of euphoria (7 to 8 seconds).
- ❍ Intramuscular injection produces a relatively slow onset of euphoria (5 to 8 minutes).
- ❍ Sniffed or smoked, peak effects are usually felt within 10 to 15 minutes.
- ❍ All three forms of heroin administration are addictive.

• • •

Above all, don't share needles

Whatever the reason for using needles, it's important always to use a clean, new needle each time and never to share needles with anyone. It's better to bring two fresh needles and give one away than to share one needle. If you can't get clean needles, clean them yourself using household bleach (specific details on how to clean needles are discussed in Day 6).

IN A SENTENCE:

> *Substance abuse begins with a genetic tendency but quickly turns into addiction with continued use.*

learning

Fixing Addiction

ASK YOURSELF: Is getting high more important than staying healthy?

If you answered "no," you are fortunate. Fixing addiction issues will probably improve the outcome of HIV. If you have advanced HIV, you might decide to treat the virus and the addiction simultaneously. Keep in mind that each condition on its own can be difficult at first.

It's possible to let your addiction go untreated while beginning HIV treatment, but your addiction may influence how well you respond to treatment, especially over the long term. Impaired thinking will reduce your ability to take the HIV medications properly over time. Impaired thinking and compulsive behaviors put you at a higher risk for other problems. Finally, substance abuse is hard on your body, which is already taxed by HIV.

Treating one condition may help with many

Fixing imbalances in your brain will probably help control several different compulsive behaviors, if that's any consolation. You will probably relapse a few times, that's usually the case. You might need a structured inpatient environment at first. Sometimes, it helps to get away from your everyday world.

Treatment for drug addiction works best in specialized treatment facilities or mental health clinics. Because drug abuse and addiction are major public health problems, a large portion of drug treatment is funded by local, state, and federal government funds. Private and employer health insurance may provide coverage for treatment of drug addiction and its medical consequences.

If you have HIV, the chances are good you'll find free addiction treatment. It's odd, but society is more willing to pay for addiction treatment for people with HIV so they don't spread the virus. Makes sense. What ultimately matters is that you get help for addiction.

Can't decide if you're addicted or not? Then test the waters and learn more about addiction to decide for yourself if you have a problem. You can start by calling the addiction hotline listed on page 274. If you have access to the Internet, there's a lot of information to be found—some of it good and some of it bad. Consider attending a twelve-step meeting. Some meetings are open to anyone. You can also find local AIDS organizations, which will point you to local meetings (see resource guide on page 275).

Checklist: You know you're hooked when...

- ○ A hit of this and a drink of that at one time was enough to hit the spot. These days, however, you crave two or three hits of this and maybe a six-pack of that.
- ○ You drink to ease your hangover. Have you ever joked about having "a hair of the dog that bit you"?
- ○ You run short of substances sooner than you planned. You could swear you just refilled that prescription for tranquilizers, and already they're gone.
- ○ You try to quit or cut down and it never seems to work out.
- ○ You spend a lot of time waiting for your dealer friend or driving across town for God-knows-what.
- ○ All your friends are the ones who really have addiction issues.
- ○ You know it's a problem, but you just keep doing it.

Nicotine is safer than tobacco

Tired of people telling you to quit smoking? Here's a way to quit without really quitting. The addictive chemical in cigarettes is nicotine, which by itself generally does not cause cancer. Burning tobacco and sucking the smoke into your lungs is the prime culprit associated with cancer. Here's the secret; you can still get your fix of nicotine without ever lighting a cigarette.

Nicotine replacement therapy keeps the nicotine flowing, but without inhaling tobacco smoke. This gives you a chance to break the habit of smoking cigarettes. Down the road, and when you're ready, you can wean yourself off the nicotine.

Nicotine replacement comes in the form of a patch applied to the skin, several flavors of gum, lozenges (not as tasty as the gum, but still does the job), and inhalers that look and taste like real cigarettes. Even nicotine-spiked lollipops can be had from the right pharmacist.

Nicotine replacement works best in the first days and months of quitting smoking. Over the long term, behavioral techniques and self-help groups produce better long-term outcomes. Behavioral techniques and self-help groups help to change your thinking or shift your perspective, teaching your old brain a few new tricks.

The combination of nicotine replacement and behavioral techniques is probably the best choice if you want to quit smoking for good.

Detox is not addiction treatment

Medically speaking, "detoxification" is a process where a person is carefully withdrawn from an addicting substance. This usually happens under the care of a physician, perhaps in an inpatient or outpatient setting.

Detox is the first step of treating drug addiction. It eases physical symptoms directly related to stopping the substance, but it doesn't fix the underlying cause of addiction. Detox is most effective in combination with an addiction treatment program.

Medicine is available for detoxification from opiates, nicotine, benzodiazepines, alcohol, barbiturates, and other sedatives. In some cases, detox is best handled in a medical setting. Withdrawal can be dangerous or fatal.

Double-action treatment for addiction works best

Eventually something will happen that makes you want to quit. There are several proven and reliable tools for putting the brakes on addiction. The tools are most effective when they are combined:

MEDICATIONS
- Nicotine replacement
- Alcohol antagonist treatment
- Antidepressants for co-occurring symptoms

○ Narcotic antagonist treatment
○ Agonist maintenance treatment

Behavioral
 ○ Counseling
 ○ Psychotherapy
 ○ Self-help groups

Principles of effective addiction treatment

The ultimate goal of all substance addiction treatment is to help to achieve lasting abstinence. Immediate goals are to (1) reduce your drug use, (2) improve your functioning, and (3) minimize medical and social complications.

According to the National Institute on Drug Abuse, drug addiction treatment should include the following thirteen principles.

1. **No single treatment is appropriate for all individuals.** You and your genes are unique. What works for the guy down the street might not work for you.
2. **Treatment needs to be easily available.** You might change your mind if finding treatment is a hassle.
3. **Treatment should help all of you, not just your drug use.** You might need assistance with medical, psychological, social, vocational, or legal issues.
4. **Assess often and modify when necessary.** Your doctor might try varying combinations of services and treatment components during the course of treatment and recovery.
5. **Give addiction treatment time to work.** Research suggests that a minimum of three months is needed for most. People usually leave treatment prematurely.
6. **Individual and/or group counseling is critical.** In counseling, you discuss motivation, tricks to resist drugs, and replacing drug activities with nondrug activities.
7. **Medications are an important element of treatment.** Medications such as methadone and levo-alphaacetylmethadol (LAAM) are effective in helping people who are addicted to heroin or other opiates. Naltrexone is also an effective medication for some opiate addicts and some patients with co-occurring alcohol dependence.

8. **Treat addiction and coexisting mood disorders in an integrated way.** Your doctor should assess you for other mood disorders such as anxiety or depression.
9. **Medical detoxification is only the first stage of addiction treatment.** Detox alone is rarely sufficient to help addicts achieve long-term abstinence.
10. **Treatment does not need to be voluntary to be effective.** You might need to be forced into treatment.
11. **Possible drug use during treatment is a concern.** Urinalysis and other tests can help you withstand urges to relapse.
12. **Address HIV and hep C in addiction treatment.** Counseling also can help you manage your health better.
13. **Recovery from drug addiction is a long-term process, often with relapses.** Don't get discouraged if you relapse a few times.

Medicine can help relieve withdrawal symptoms

Of course, taking a drug to stop taking a drug may seem strange at first. But studies show that you can improve favorable outcomes for drug addiction treatment by using certain medications. The medications will work better if they're used with counseling, therapy, and careful monitoring. In order for the drugs to work, however, you have to take them as prescribed. Here are some of the drugs used to treat addiction:

Agonist Maintenance Treatment, for opiate addicts, is usually conducted in outpatient settings, often called methadone treatment programs. These programs use a long-acting synthetic opiate medication given by mouth, usually methadone or LAAM to prevent opiate withdrawal, block the effects of illicit opiate use, and decrease opiate craving. Patients stabilized on methadone or LAAM can function normally.

People stabilized on opiate agonists are better able to participate in counseling and other behavioral interventions. The best, most effective opiate agonist maintenance programs include individual and/or group counseling along with other needed medical, psychological, and social services.

Antagonist Treatment blocks all the euphoria and effects of self-administered opiates. Because narcotic antagonists don't let you get "high" from opiates, it's hoped that the compulsion to use will be decreased. A drug called naltrexone is often used for this purpose. Naltrexone is also used to help treat alcohol dependence.

Buprenorphine is an alternative to methadone for treating opiate addiction. Buprenorphine is a partial opioid agonist. At low doses, it behaves as an agonist, and at high doses, as either an agonist or antagonist, depending on the circumstances. In 2002, buprenorphine hydrochloride (Subutex) was approved in the United States for the treatment of opioid dependence and is available by prescription.

Antabuse is the trade name for the drug tetraethylthiuram disulfide, used in the treatment of alcoholism. Also called sulfiram, Antabuse is non-toxic, but it alters the metabolism of alcohol in the body, making it impossible for you to get drunk without experiencing severe discomfort.

Today's drug rehab is not your mother's drug rehab

Addiction medicine has come a long way in the last twenty years. Research has shown that combining addiction medicine with behavioral therapy yields the best results. In some cases, people may need to "take a vacation" from their regular routine. Some people call this "rehab." Whatever you call it, here's a few options:

Therapeutic communities are highly structured programs in which patients stay at a residence, typically for six to twelve months. This approach is best for people with relatively long histories of drug dependence, involvement in serious criminal activities, and impaired social functioning. Many therapeutic communities are quite comprehensive and can include employment training and other support services on site.

Short-term residential programs are sometimes referred to as chemical dependency clinics. These programs involve a three to six week inpatient treatment phase followed by extended outpatient therapy or participation in twelve-step self-help groups, such as Narcotics Anonymous or Cocaine Anonymous.

Methadone maintenance programs are usually more successful at retaining clients with opiate dependence than are therapeutic communities, which in turn are more successful than outpatient programs that provide psychotherapy and counseling.

Outpatient drug-free treatment does not include medications and encompasses a wide variety of programs for patients who visit a clinic at regular intervals. Most of the programs involve individual or group counseling. This is a reasonable option for non-opiate addiction. Some outpatient programs treat people who have medical or mood disorders in addition to addiction.

Community Reinforcement Approach is an intensive twenty-four week outpatient therapy for treatment of cocaine addiction. The treatment goals are twofold:

○ To achieve cocaine abstinence long enough for you to learn new life skills that will help sustain abstinence.

○ To reduce alcohol consumption if drinking is associated with cocaine. Be prepared to submit urine samples two or three times each week.

Self-help groups

The best-known twelve-step program is Alcoholics Anonymous (AA). The twelve-step approach to recovery is better known, and AA is more widely available. For this reason, it is a critical part of recovery for many addicts. If the twelve-step is not your dance, there are other self-help groups such as Rational Recovery or Women for Sobriety.

The twelve-step philosophy is not intrinsically related to alcohol. The AA model has spawned related recovery programs including

○ Narcotics Anonymous (NA)
○ Cocaine Anonymous (CA)
○ Overeaters Anonymous (OA)
○ Sexual Compulsives Anonymous (SCA).

All adhere to the same basic philosophy of AA. Twelve-step ideology is built on twelve steps, or lessons, organized from basic to advance. The approach eventually suggests that members recognize the existence of a higher power.

AA at a glance

Most drug addiction treatment programs encourage people to participate in a self-help group during and after formal treatment. You can find an AA meeting almost anytime or anywhere, if you know where to look. In the United States, there are meetings in every state and every major city. Many larger cities provide telephone numbers to call for specific times and locations. In larger cities, some AA meetings may deal specifically with HIV and addiction. To find out more information about AA meetings, you can try calling an AIDS service organization (see the resource guide on page 275), a state HIV hotline, or look online at http://www.aa.org.

Here's what to expect:

○ At an AA meeting, members sit in a room and talk about their experiences with drinking problems.

- ○ They talk, sometimes, about the Twelve Steps.
- ○ The format varies; often there's one speaker but other times everyone takes a turn speaking.

Here's what *not* to expect:

- ○ initial motivation to recover
- ○ religious preaching
- ○ medical or psychological services

One minor detail to keep in mind about AA meetings: sometimes discussion of HIV is frowned upon—except at the specific AA meetings that deal directly with HIV issues. "I tried to go to twelve-step meetings and share about HIV when I first got clean, but they told me it was an 'outside issue,'" says Rosetta M., who is HIV-positive and a recovering addict. "At first, I couldn't understand it."

"Underneath it all, I think that there are people with HIV in the [A.A. and other twelve-step] rooms and they are not sharing about it, so they resent when somebody comes in and shares about HIV. Or they are still engaging in [risk] behaviors, and they don't want you to rain on their parade. I think there's a lot of reasons and a lot of environments that people don't want to hear about HIV."

Sex addiction is neither "sex" nor "addiction"

There's a thin line between addiction and compulsion. Addiction is a physical need for some substance, while compulsion is a desire to do some behavior. The zinger is that some behaviors trigger dopamine in ways similar to those seen with substance addiction. It's not clear yet if certain behaviors spike dopamine, which causes an addiction-like state in the brain.

Either way, "sex addiction" is how most people refer to "sexual compulsion." Obsessive-compulsive behavior may include preoccupation with finding sex, soliciting prostitutes, or whatever. Sexual compulsion is being recognized as a major social problem with similarities to alcohol and drugs.

If particular patterns of sexual behavior start to feel "unmanageable," you're probably inclined toward sexual compulsion. You might feel out of control at times. At other times, you might feel shame and self-loathing. Still, you keep doing it.

Obsessive-compulsive behaviors are treatable. Two effective treatments are psychotherapy and medication with a serotonin reuptake inhibitor.

Doctors often combine these approaches. Self-help groups complement and extend the effects of treatment.

One popular group is called Sexual Compulsive Anonymous (SCA). Based on the twelve-step model, SCA meetings are like AA meetings, but instead of alcohol, the problem is compulsive behavior related to sex. Meetings are open to anyone who wants to recover from sexual compulsion, regardless of sexual orientations.

The main difference between SCA and AA is that while you can abstain from alcohol, abstaining from sex is not the answer for most. The focus of SCA is not to repress sexuality, but to help you express it in ways that don't steal your time and energy—or place you in legal jeopardy. Each member develops a "sexual recovery plan," defining what sexual sobriety means for himself or herself.

IN A SENTENCE:

Consider treating substance abuse, addiction, and compulsive behavior to improve your odds for successful HIV treatment down the road.

Nutrition and Exercise

AMERICANS ARE getting fat and people with HIV are no different. Between 1991 and 2000, obesity among the general population increased by 60 percent, with one in five being obese and one in three being overweight. At the same time, almost one in four Americans with HIV are dieting to lose weight.

Half the Fat of Regular People

HIV population compared to the general population

GENERAL POPULATION
Two in three—overweight
Two in five—obese

PEOPLE WITH HIV
One in three—overweight
One in ten—obese

If people with HIV were a snack food, they'd be considered "Lite" by the USDA. But being half as fat as the general population is not saying much. Clearly, the old image of people with HIV as being undernourished and emaciated no longer holds true. Since the introduction of the new HIV treatments, the prevalence of malnutrition among the HIV population has fallen by almost 50 percent. Even more encouraging is a 77 percent decrease in the prevalence of "wasting," a specific medical condition characterized by "unintentional loss of more than 10 percent of body weight." It's certainly no mistake that the decrease of wasting rates is almost identical to the decrease of rates of "full-blown" AIDS. The lesson: less AIDS, less wasting.

A recent study showed that the rates of wasting were still significant among people with HIV. The study also showed that the rates of obesity among the same population were more common than the rates of wasting:

- 6 percent—wasting
- 34 percent—overweight
- 9 percent—obese

The researchers were careful to note that HIV treatment itself was not the cause of being overweight or obese. Instead, they concluded that "dietary and lifestyle advice" should be included as a component of HIV treatment.

At the same time, people who are taking HIV treatment are increasingly reporting that their levels of cholesterol and triglycerides, both of which are special types of fat found in the blood, are climbing. Cholesterol and triglycerides are associated with obesity, diabetes, high blood pressure, and heart problems—all of which are also being reported among people with HIV. (There's a related but somewhat different condition called **lipodystrophy**, which is discussed in Month 7).

What does all this mean for you? It means that having HIV doesn't get you off the hook when it comes to nutritious eating and honest exercise. In fact, healthy eating and exercise are very likely to be more important because you have the virus. Let's face it, if you plan on living a long time with HIV, you'll need to eat well and exercise.

Television, bookstores, magazine racks, and the Internet are brimming with the latest "news" on fitness and diet fads. Some of the advice is good, but most of it seems conflicting, confusing, and probably even misleading.

Don't let this noise distract you from the time-tested, proven, safe, and sound principles of fitness:

1. If you're below a healthy weight, you should eat nutritiously and exercise more often to gain or maintain weight.

2. If you're overweight, you should eat nutritiously in smaller portions and exercise more often to lose weight.

It really is that simple.

What "they" say about nutrition and HIV is wrong

Fortunately, it's a new ball game when it comes to HIV. Unfortunately, the conventional wisdom about nutrition for people with HIV is stuck in the 1990s. Doctors don't manage HIV like they did back then. In the same way, you shouldn't be eating like you're on death's door—unless, of course, your goal is to be on death's door.

If you've been to an HIV doctor or an HIV clinic, you've probably seen all the colorful brochures that claim wasting is still a major problem and that the latest pill or steroid can help you "gain weight." What these "pharmaceutical-sponsored" brochures fail to mention is that their claims are based on old research.

The advice offered by these brochures is based on research done in the 1990s. Back then, people with HIV were generally sicker, had higher viral loads and lower T-cells. At the time, the nutritional needs of these people were very different.

In the 1990s, treatments and a booming business emerged to help people with HIV combat the physical deterioration that's associated with AIDS. Pharmaceutical companies developed a variety of new products. Dieticians and physical therapists began selling their services to people with AIDS. Makers of nutritional and herbal supplements proliferated. "Crisis management" was the mantra of the times.

Today, however, the crisis is over and the focus should be on maintaining health for the long term. Look carefully at those brochures—they're ultimately trying to sell you something or "prime their market." There's a lot of money in the business of prescriptions or supplmenets to manipulate body weight.

Think about nutrition and HIV in one of two ways

There are new ways to think about HIV. On one hand, there's "uncontrolled HIV," which means that the virus is running rampant, gobbling up T-cells, and generally making a mess of your body. People with moderate-to-high viral load levels, depleted immune systems, or both, have uncontrolled HIV. This was the case with many people in the 1990s. On the other hand, there's "controlled HIV." In this state, HIV treatments are keeping the virus in check. People with controlled HIV have very low viral loads that may be below the limit of detection.

A critical distinction, however, is *how* the virus is being controlled. If you have a low viral load and you're not taking HIV treatment, it means your immune system is working double duty. For the purposes of nutrition, let's refer to that scenario as "uncontrolled HIV." If you are taking HIV treatment, and your viral load is very low or undetectable, that's controlled HIV. Your immune system doesn't need to work as hard, and your nutritional needs may change as well.

Imagine this: You're in a log cabin on a very cold night. To stay warm, you find some wood logs and stoke up a fire in the fireplace. The cabin warms up to a nice cozy temperature.

In this metaphor, think of the cabin as your body, the fireplace as your immune system, and the wood logs as the food you eat. In your cabin, you throw a log on the fire every few hours to keep the temperature comfortable, just as you would eat three times a day to remain healthy. This is the normal state of healthy human bodies.

Now imagine that someone throws a rock through a window in your cabin. This is a little like getting infected with HIV. Of course, the cabin may stay warm at first, but you know it won't last long because the heat is escaping through the window faster than the fireplace can make more heat. What do you do? You have two choices: start tossing more logs in the fireplace more often, or patch the window.

Back in the 1990s, people with HIV did not have the right treatments to "patch the hole in the window." So the obvious choice—back then—was to start throwing logs on the fire. At the time, researchers and nutritionists recommended that people with HIV eat more food, especially rich, fatty food to fuel their broken immune systems. After all, the virus and the immune system were battling fiercely. People with HIV ate up to provide the fuel, as food, for both the virus and the immune system. "Eat!" the researchers told people with HIV, sometimes suggesting they take in double the calories and protein. It made sense back then.

Now imagine you're back in the cabin with a broken window and you haven't gotten around to patching the window. Instead, you decide to burn logs more often to keep the heat at a comfortable level. But, you also know there's only a limited number of trees to burn and eventually you'll run short.

Finally, you decide it's time to patch the window. In this example, patching the window is like taking HIV treatment: You fix the underlying problem. However, after you fix the window, would you continue to throw logs on the

Diabetes and HIV

WHY PEOPLE with HIV should care:

○ Diabetes risk increased threefold in HIV-positive women treated with anti-HIV drugs called protease inhibitors.
○ Research has shown increases in the incidence of diabetes among HIV-positives, compared to HIV-negatives.
○ Among people with HIV, 34 percent are overweight and 9 percent are obese.
○ Weight gain of eleven to eighteen pounds doubles your risk of developing type 2 diabetes.
○ About 80 percent of people with diabetes are overweight or obese.
○ One-third of people with diabetes don't know that they have it.

WHAT IS DIABETES?

Diabetes is a disorder of metabolism—the way our bodies use digested food for growth and energy. Most of the food we eat gets converted into glucose, which is the body's main source of energy. Cells can only absorb glucose when insulin, a hormone made by the pancreas, is present.

When you have diabetes, you don't produce or respond to insulin. With diabetes, glucose builds up in the blood, overflows into the urine, and passes out of the body. Thus, your body loses its main source of fuel.

SYMPTOMS OF DIABETES

People with diabetes might not have symptoms. When they do, the most common symptoms are

○ excessive thirst
○ excessive hunger
○ excessive urination
○ unintended weight loss
○ tingling or numbness in feet or hands
○ sores that are slow to heal
○ dry itchy skin

DIABETES IS PREVENTABLE

A large body of evidence shows that certain types of diabetes can be prevented or reversed with good nutrition and exercise.

fire at the same rate? Of course not. The cabin would get too hot. In the same way, if you continue to eat as the researchers told the HIV-positive throughout the 1990s, you'd get fat and put yourself at other health risks such as heart disease and diabetes.

"I would treat individuals with HIV who are on [HIV] therapy as high-risk cardiovascular patients—without a doubt," says Anthony S. Fauci, M.D., director of the National Institute of Allergy and Infectious Diseases. "In other words, I would say to assume that you have a forty-five-year-old father who died of a myocardial infarction, your cholesterol is very high, and your mother had diabetes—even though it might not be the case. You have to treat yourself like that. You have to be careful with diet. You have to make sure that you don't fuel an engine of risk that you unfortunately have."

STATES OF THE VIRUS: "ON" OR "OFF"
Eating for *controlled* and *uncontrolled* HIV are two very different situations.

UNCONTROLLED HIV
○   moderate-to-high viral load levels
○   low T-cells

CONTROLLED HIV
○   very low viral levels
○   "undetectable" (less than 40 copies)

Basics of a healthy diet

The USDA food pyramid is a reasonable diet if you adhere to reasonable portion sizes. But who does? At the same time, fast food and the availability of processed foods—cookies, cake, chips, and soda—have merged to make us fat.

Consensus is building among health professionals that an eating style derived from the Mediterranean region may be healthier than the typical American diet. Sometimes called the Mediterranean Diet, this eating style has been well studied because of the notably low incidence of chronic diseases and high life expectancy associated with it.

• • •

10 PRINCIPLES OF THE MEDITERRANEAN DIET

1. An abundance of food from plant sources, including fruits and vegetables, potatoes, breads and grains, beans, nuts, and seeds
2. Emphasis on a variety of minimally processed and, wherever possible, seasonally fresh and locally grown foods (which often maximizes the health-promoting micronutrient and antioxidant content of these foods)
3. Olive oil as the principal fat, replacing other fats and oils (including butter and margarine)
4. Total fat ranging from less than 25 percent to over 35 percent of energy, with saturated fat no more than 7 to 8 percent of calories
5. Daily consumption of low to moderate amounts of cheese and yogurt (low-fat and nonfat versions may be preferable)
6. Weekly consumption of low to moderate amounts of fish and poultry (recent research suggests that fish be somewhat favored over poultry), from zero to four eggs per week (including those used in cooking and baking)
7. Fresh fruit as the typical daily dessert; sweets with a significant amount of sugar (often as honey) and saturated fat consumed no more than a few times per week
8. Red meat a few times per month (recent research suggests that if red meat is eaten, its consumption should be limited to a maximum of 12 to 16 ounces per month; where the flavor is acceptable, lean versions may be preferable)
9. Regular physical activity at a level that promotes a healthy weight, fitness, and well-being
10. Moderate consumption of wine, normally with meals; about one to two glasses per day for men and one glass per day for women (wine should be considered optional and avoided when consumption would put the individual or others at risk)

In a similar way, the American Cancer Society has developed guidelines for nutrition and cancer prevention. The key principles of this diet include the following:

○ Choose most of the foods you eat from plant sources
○ Limit your intake of high-fat foods, particularly from animal sources
○ Be physically active. Achieve and maintain a healthy weight

If you do nothing else, do this:
○ Eat more fruits and vegetables every day

Vitamins and supplements are not fruits and vegetables

People who don't like vegetables may try to get by with vitamins. This isn't necessarily a bad idea; it's just not a good one. Studies show that 75 percent of people with HIV use some form of alternative medicine including megavitamins and supplements. But studies done of the general population are also beginning to show that the health benefits of a nutritious diet are not explained by vitamins and supplements alone.

The missing link may be certain substances—besides vitamins and minerals—found only in plants. One name for these substances is phytochemicals, which represent thousands of different components in plant foods.

Phytochemicals are not considered "essential" nutrients. But eating an abundance of phytochemicals from various fruits and vegetables has been associated with the prevention and/or treatment of at least four of the leading causes of death in the United States—cancer, heart disease, diabetes, and high blood pressure.

The specific phytochemical content of different fruits and vegetables tends to vary by color, and each has unique functions. Some phytochemicals act as antioxidants, some protect and regenerate essential nutrients, and others work to deactivate cancer-causing substances.

The top ten food groups that provide the most vitamins, minerals, and phytochemicals include

- Red, yellow, and orange fruits
- Red, yellow, and orange vegetables
- Cruciferous and leafy green vegetables
- Mushrooms
- Sea vegetables
- Garlic and similar plants
- Whole grains
- Beans and other legumes
- Soy and soy products
- Nuts and seeds

. . .

Diet, Exercise, and HIV: A Case Study

RESEARCHERS AT Tufts University reported the results of a forty-four-year-old man who was assigned to an intensive diet and exercise regimen for four months. The man had been taking HIV treatment for two and a half years.

THE PROBLEM:

- ○ gained thirty pounds
- ○ experiencing "lipodystrophy," an abnormal body fat condition
- ○ lost body fat in limbs, but gained it in chest and waistline

THE DIET

- ○ consumed at least 25 grams of dietary fiber daily
- ○ 15 percent of total caloric intake from protein
- ○ 30 percent from fat
- ○ 55 percent from carbs

THE EXERCISE

- ○ cardio plus strength training
- ○ 75-minute workout sessions three times a week

THE RESULTS

- ○ lost fourteen pounds
- ○ lowered cholesterol levels
- ○ 28 percent decrease in body fat
- ○ 52 percent decrease in intra-abdominal fat—fat around the internal organs
- ○ maintained improvements after one year on the regimen

THE LESSON FOR PEOPLE WITH HIV

Researchers concluded that lifestyle solutions—not just pharmaceuticals—can be a powerful treatment for lipodystrophy and many other conditions.

Exercise is good for your heart and head, not your T-cells

It's not true that exercise helps fight HIV. Research has consistently shown that exercise has no effect on T-cells or viral load. End of story.

One caveat: More and more metabolic conditions are being reported among people with HIV. It's not yet clear if these conditions stem from a damaged immune system, the virus itself, or HIV treatments. Some researchers suggest it's a complicated mix of them all.

The conditions include

- fat redistribution (lipodystrophy)
- loss of fat in the extremities (lipoatrophy)
- excess of fat around the internal organs (severe visceral adiposity)
- high cholesterol and triglycerides (lipid abnormalities)
- insulin abnormalities (hyperinsulinemia)
- unusually high blood sugar (hyperglycemia)
- weak bones (osteopenia)

Whatever the true cause, all of these conditions are becoming more common in the HIV population. It puts people with HIV at a higher risk for diabetes, pancreatitis, bone disorders, and heart disease. Exercise is proving to do more than "not hurt." It may actually help. Research is showing that exercise reduces and sometimes eliminates—and may even prevent—these conditions. After all, who wants to survive HIV only to have a heart attack later in life?

But wait, there's more. In addition to just helping your body, exercise helps your mind. Research has shown it helps people with HIV cope better with the stresses of life. One study showed that people who were "regular exercisers" had less anxiety and depression after receiving an HIV-positive diagnosis. The researchers concluded that "exercise appeared to provide a 'buffer' to the psychological stress" of living with the virus.

Cope better, and you'll make better health decisions over the long haul. Make better decisions over the long haul, and you'll spin the odds of good fortune in your favor.

• • •

"Inner" fat is worse than garden-variety fat.

The most dangerous kind of fat is not what hangs over your belt. The danger lies deep within the belly, behind the stomach muscles. It's called "intra-abdominal fat," and as it grows, it wraps around your internal organs and can strangle them. Sometimes, this fat infiltrates your liver.

Inner fat makes people look like the shape of an apple versus the shape of a pear. Among the general population, this particular distribution of fat is more common among older people. People with HIV are more prone to this inner fat for reasons related to the severity of immune depletion and length of time on HIV treatments. Either way, pinching an inch can't tell you how much inner fat lurks on the inside.

Some of the disease risks of excessive intra-abdominal fat:

- ○ Heart disease
- ○ High blood pressure
- ○ Stroke
- ○ Type 2 diabetes
- ○ Certain forms of cancer, including uterine, breast, and colon

Exercise shrinks inner fat

"Exercise is amazing," says Anthony S. Fauci, M.D., "Exercise does so many good things for you. It keeps your blood pressure down. It keeps your resting heart rate down. It gives you a level of endorphins that just makes you feel better generally."

Besides making you feel better, moderate exercise can reduce intra-abdominal fat. Researchers at Tufts University studied HIV-positive people, some of whom were taking HIV treatments, while others were not. The researchers found that exercise increased physical functioning, led to weight loss, decreased stomach girth, and reduced fatigue. However, there was no difference in T-cells or virus levels between groups.

A related study found body composition, bone density, and lipid, insulin, and glucose levels all appeared to improve with exercise. The researchers are finding a few guidelines to combat intra-abdominal fat. They include:

- ○ moderate-intensity cardio workout
- ○ resistance training (weight lifting)
- ○ eating well to achieve a healthy weight

Cardio exercise makes your heart beat faster

When you exercise, your heart beats faster to meet the demand for more blood and oxygen by the muscles of the body. The more intense the activity, the faster your heart will beat. Therefore, monitoring your heart rate during exercise can be an excellent way to monitor exercise intensity. According to the American Council on Exercise, the target is to work your heart to about 50 to 80 percent of its capacity.

Maximal Heart Rate: This number is related to your age. As we grow older, our hearts start to beat a little more slowly. To estimate your maximal heart rate, simply subtract your age from the number 220.

Target Heart-Rate Zone: This is the number of beats per minute at which your heart should be beating during cardio exercise.

CALCULATING A CARDIO PLAN

Bob is thirty-six years old and he wants to find his target heart rate.

Step 1

220 minus 36 is 184. This number, 184, is Bob's maximal heart rate.

Step 2

To find Bob's 50 percent heart rate, divide by two. For Bob, that's 92. The number 92 is the minimum number of beats per minute he needs to earn cardio benefits.

Step 3

To find Bob's 80 percent heart rate, use the chart below.

Age:	20	30	40	50	60	70
50%	100	95	90	85	80	75
80%	160	152	144	136	128	120

Now, calculate your target heart rate. However, don't forget the target heart-rate zone is just an estimate. If when you exercise, it feels too hard, it probably is too hard. The time you should keep your heart beating in the target zone depends on many factors.

If you're keeping a health journal (see Day 7 for a reminder on setting up a health journal), you'll want to write down your target zone and track over time how often you reach the zone.

New physical activity targets included among the National Academy of Sciences Institute of Medicine guidelines say that people should get sixty minutes daily of moderate exercise, such as walking at four miles per hour. The amount recommended by the U.S. Health and Human Services is thirty minutes of moderate exercise each day. The message: exercise between thirty and sixty minutes every day.

HERE ARE A FEW EXAMPLES OF A CARDIO WORKOUT:
- playing volleyball for 45 minutes
- walking 1¾ miles in 35 minutes (20 min/mile)
- bicycling 5 miles in 30 minutes
- dancing fast (social) for 30 minutes
- walking 2 miles in 30 minutes (15 min/mile)
- swimming laps for 20 minutes
- basketball (playing a game) for 15-20 minutes
- bicycling 4 miles in 15 minutes
- running 1½ miles in 15 minutes (10 min/mile)
- shoveling snow for 15 minutes

Strength training builds muscle, tendons, and ligaments

Even if vanity drives you to resistance training, that's fine. Think about it: the vanity benefits come from looking healthy. More resistance training can help you look healthy and be healthy. The benefits won't only be in terms of muscle. Your bones will benefit too. Your bones will line up better because of stronger connective tissue, called tendons and ligaments. With better tendons and ligaments, you're less prone to injury.

If you're serious about resistance training, find a trainer

Everyone can benefit from a little guidance from a certified personal trainer, says Timothy M. Brewi, a personal trainer and editor of *HIV Fitness Guidelines*. Even advanced fitness enthusiasts can benefit from a check-in with a trainer to correct poor exercise habits, such as a stale exercise routine.

"As for a specific exercise plan, there's no one-size-fits-all routine," said Brewi. "Generally, a well-balanced plan includes aerobic exercise, resistance exercise, and stretching. But many other disciplines, such as yoga and

Everything You Ever Want to Know about Exercise and HIV

YOU DON'T have to go to a gym to strength train. You can keep weights in your house or even use soup cans (full, no cheating). If you want more information about how, visit http://www.hivfitness.org. Health professionals with HIV experience operate the Web site. The group's philosophy is that while exercise may improve your physical appearance, it makes little sense to risk health with dangerous exercises, extreme diets, expensive supplements, or excessive drug use.

KEY ELEMENTS OF STRENGTH TRAINING
American Council on Exercise

○ Vary your exercises to work all the major muscle groups. Neglecting certain groups can lead to strength imbalances and postural difficulties.

○ One set of 8–12 repetitions, working the muscle to the point of fatigue, is usually sufficient.

○ Breathe normally throughout the exercise.

○ Lower the resistance with a slow, controlled cadence throughout the full range of motion.

○ Lifting the weight to a count of two and lowering it to a count of three or four is effective.

○ When you are able to perform 12 repetitions of an exercise correctly (without cheating), increase the amount of resistance by 5 to 10 percent to continue safe progress.

○ Aim to exercise each muscle group at least two times per week, with a minimum of two days of rest between workouts.

○ Training more frequently or adding more sets may lead to slightly greater gains, but the small added benefit may not be worth the extra time and effort (not to mention the added risk of injury).

○ Use machines and free weights to provide exercise variety, which is important for both psychological and physiological reasons. Variety not only reduces boredom, but also provides subtle exercise differences that will enhance progress.

pilates, may suit someone's activity preference and enhance their state of fitness. The key is to find activities that you enjoy enough to keep doing on a regular basis. A good exercise plan doesn't necessarily have to include working out at the gym."

IN A SENTENCE:

> *A nutritious diet with more fruits and vegetables and regular cardio and strength training are more important when you have HIV.*

learning

Why and When to Treat HIV

HAVE YOU ever received a bill in the mail and set it aside? Maybe you thought, "I'll deal with it later." Maybe you didn't even think about it. That is, until your phone went dead because you forgot to pay the bill on time. Then you scrambled to pay the bill—along with late fees.

Treating HIV is a little like paying bills. You can ignore or "set aside" learning about HIV treatment. Sometimes, that's a reasonable way to cope with a tough situation. In fact, a large study of people who were newly diagnosed with HIV found that most delay seeing a doctor for a year or more. But at the same time, another study found that people with HIV who use "denial" progress to AIDS faster than those who don't. The point is, many people don't want to think about HIV—but this can make things worse for you.

In the short run, ignoring or denying your health situation might be what you need to get through the next few months. But, like everything else in life, *you will have to deal with your situation—either by your own choice or by being forced to deal with it*. Dealing with things sooner rather than later always turns out to be a little better.

Your T-cells and viral load are what they are. Denial and wishful thinking will not change your situation. If your T-cells are low or your viral load is high, you'll need to make some important decisions sooner rather than later. If your T-cells are high and viral load is low, you have the luxury of more time to consider your options.

Either way, moving past denial doesn't mean you must decide everything today; it means having an open mind, being receptive to information, and honestly assessing what is happening in your life. If you can do this, you're ready to start.

The benefits of learning about HIV treatment and becoming a smarter patient are immense. They include:

○ **living longer**—studies have shown that denial is associated with decreased survival.
○ **living better**—knowing your treatment options will increase your chances of picking a successful yet convenient treatment.
○ **enjoying better treatments in the future**—HIV treatment gets better every year; you can position yourself now to take advantage of treatment and strategies down the road.

Treating HIV is always your decision

At times, it may seem like your doctor is pushing treatment on you. Depending on your doctor and your health situation, this might be true. However, your doctor has probably witnessed the damage that AIDS can do. You've probably never seen anyone with "full-blown" AIDS. It is horrendous.

Untreated, HIV will progress to AIDS in almost everyone. During the first few years, you will probably feel fine, but the virus and your immune system will be fiercely battling. With time and as your immune system is depleted, you might start to feel tired, your lymph nodes might become swollen or painful, and you'll probably notice small things like recurrent rashes, diarrhea, or yeast infections in your mouth.

Eventually, you will get a major infection like pneumonia. You'll become very sick. You'll get scared. Then, you'll probably recover and feel better for some time. But you will get sick again. This time, it might be with something new, like skin cancer or a bacterial infection of the brain. You'll vomit and have uncontrollable diarrhea. Your muscles will shrink and you might go blind. If you're lucky, you won't have too much pain. Eventually, you will die.

This scenario is what you and your doctor are trying to prevent. The way to stay healthy is to preserve your immune system. The way to preserve your immune system is to reduce your viral load. And, currently, the only way to reduce your viral load is by HIV drug treatment.

AIDS-Defining Opportunistic Infections

THE CDC uses specific criteria for determining when a person living with HIV progresses to AIDS. If a person falls below 200 T-cells, theoretically that person has progressed to AIDS. But that threshold is for categorizing purposes. Another way that the CDC defines AIDS is having HIV *plus* one of several opportunistic infections. They include:

Bacterial Infections
- Mycobacterium avium complex (MAC)
- Salmonellosis
- Syphilis and Neurosyphilis
- Tuberculosis (TB)

Malignancies (Cancers)
- Anal dysplasia/cancer
- Cervical dysplasia/cancer
- Kaposi's Sarcoma (KS)
- Lymphomas

Viral Infections
- Cytomegalovirus (CMV)
- Herpes simplex virus (oral and genital herpes)
- Herpes zoster virus (shingles)
- Human papiloma virus (a.k.a. HPV, genital warts, anal/cervical dysplasia/cancer)
- Molluscum contagiosum
- Oral hairy leukoplakia (OHL)
- Progressive multifocal leukoencephalopathy (PML)

Fungal Infections
- Aspergillosis
- **Candidiasis** (thrush, yeast infection)
- Coccidioidomycosis
- Cryptococcal meningitis
- Histoplasmosis

Protozoal Infections
- Cryptosporidiosis
- Isosporiasis
- Microsporidiosis
- *Pneumocystis carinii* pneumonia (PCP)
- Toxoplasmosis

Neurological Conditions
- AIDS dementia complex
- Peripheral neuropathy

HIV treatment is almost always effective in reducing viral load. Without the burden of fighting the virus, your immune system will begin to rebuild itself. You will probably experience a gradual increase in T-cells, sometimes to normal levels. This increase in T-cells is what will keep you healthy and alive.

Treatment guidelines and strategies have emerged to help patients and doctors better understand the risks of HIV treatment versus the risks of not treating the virus. Physicians, researchers, and consumers in conjunction with the US Department of Health and Human Services (DHHS) developed one set of treatment guidelines. HIV researchers and physicians in conjunction with the International AIDS Society-USA (IAS), a nonprofit physician education organization, created another set of guidelines, which often focuses more on areas where there is controversy or insufficient research for definitive approaches to care or treatment.

Taken together, both documents represent the latest thinking about HIV treatment and serve as roadmaps for people with the virus. Both documents are revised regularly—sometimes from year to year—so it's important to keep track of any major changes that might affect your decisions about treatment.

Both documents are available on the Internet. The DHHS document, called the "Guidelines for the Use of Antiretroviral Agents in HIV-Infected Adults and Adolescents," is available at http://www.aidsinfo.nih.gov/. The IAS document, called the "Updated Recommendations for the Use of Antiretroviral Therapy," is available at http://www.iasusa.org.

The following chapters incorporate information from both sets of treatment guidelines, reflecting a range of opinions. Both guidelines can be intimidating for people without medical training. To start getting a grip on the complicated—and rapidly changing—worlds of HIV treatment, it's best to slow and get a fee for the big picture first.

Goals of HIV treatment

Within the medical community, there is a consensus about the goals of HIV treatment. The primary goals include:

○ preserving your immune system
○ lowering your viral load as much as possible for as long as possible
○ minimizing side effects from treatment
○ reducing sickness and death due to HIV

T-cell count tests measure how far HIV disease has progressed

T-cell (CD4+) tests are normally reported as the number of cells in a cubic millimeter of blood, or mm^3. There is some disagreement about the normal range for T-cell counts, but normal CD4+ counts are between 500 and 1600. T-cell counts drop dramatically in people with HIV, in some cases down to zero.

The T-cell value bounces around a lot. Time of day, fatigue, and stress can affect the test results. It's best to have blood drawn at the same time of day for each T-cell test, and to use the same laboratory. Infections and vaccinations can have a large impact on your T-cell counts. So don't check your T-cells until a couple of weeks after you recover from an infection, or after you get a vaccination.

350 AND HIGHER T-CELLS

If your T-cells are above 350, your risk of progressing to AIDS within three years is relatively low. A T-cell count of 350 or higher generally means that HIV has not progressed very far. Of course, the higher the number, the better. However, when your T-cells are consistently above 350, your immune system is in relatively good shape. You should be able to fight infections fairly well.

When considering HIV treatment at this stage, you should know that some benefits have been reported, however, people with 350 or more T-cells tend to report more long-term side effects from HIV treatment. In fact, 40 percent of these people switched medications due to side effects and 20 percent discontinued treatment after two years.

Since the risk of disease progression is low, you should weigh this fact against potential risks of HIV therapy, how treatment may affect your quality of life, and how you will respond to future treatments. You should also consider your viral load (see below). For most people in this category, the risks of HIV therapy outweigh the risks of disease progression.

200 TO 350 T-CELLS

If your T-cells are between 200 and 350, your risk of progressing to AIDS is significantly higher. This means that HIV has already progressed somewhat and has done some damage to your immune system. However, this category is the gray zone of HIV treatment.

Some serious illnesses, especially tuberculosis and pneumonia, can occur when your T-cells are above 200. When considering HIV treatment, you should know that people generally respond less well to treatment when their T-cells are near 200. Some of these poor responses include:

○ slower increase in T-cells count after starting treatment
○ decreased ability to lower viral load to below the limit of detection
○ increased ability of HIV to become resistant to treatment

If your T-cells are in this range, your viral load is far more important in tipping the scales to treat or delay treatment. If your viral load is high, there's a much greater risk for progressing to AIDS.

200 OR LESS T-CELLS

If your T-cells are less than 200, this is not good. Your immune system has been severely damaged by HIV, and you may not be able to fight infections. You will need to take special medicine to prevent certain diseases (notably a certain form of pneumonia) and start HIV treatment immediately.

Studies have shown that people with HIV are more likely to die if they start HIV treatment when their T-cells are below 200, compared to starting when their T-cells are higher. HIV therapy should not be delayed if your T-cell count is below 200.

Viral load test measures how fast HIV disease is progressing

There are different techniques for measuring HIV viral load: the PCR (polymerase chain reaction) test and the bDNA (branched DNA) test. The PCR test results are often different from the bDNA results for the same sample. Because the tests are different, you should stick with the same kind of test (PCR or bDNA) to measure your viral load over time. Be sure to ask your doctor which test was used.

Viral loads are usually reported as "copies" of HIV in one milliliter of blood. The tests count up to about 1.5 million copies, and are always being improved to be more sensitive. The first bDNA test measured down to 10,000 copies. The second-generation could detect as few as 400 copies. Now there are FDA-approved tests that have a lower limit of 50 copies.

The best viral load test result is "undetectable." However, this does not mean that there is no virus in your blood; it just means that there is not enough for the test to find and count. For example, with the second-generation test, "undetectable" could mean 399 copies. "Undetectable" depends on the sensitivity of the test used.

VIRAL LOAD OF LESS THAN 50
If your viral load is less than 50 copies, many doctors will report this as "undetectable." This is great news. This means that HIV has basically been stopped in its tracks.

VIRAL LOAD OF LESS THAN 400
If your viral load is less than 400 copies, this is good news for now. This means that HIV is progressing very slowly. Some doctors may inaccurately report a viral load of less than 400 as "undetectable." Keep in mind that a viral load of less than 400 is not as good as less than 50. Be sure to ask what the lower limit of detection is for the viral load test your doctor performed.

VIRAL LOAD OF BETWEEN 400 AND 5,000
If your viral load is in between 400 and 5,000, this is not ideal, but it isn't bad news. A viral load in this range is generally considered on the low end of the scale. It means that HIV is progressing at a slow-to-moderate pace.

VIRAL LOAD OF BETWEEN 5,000 AND 30,000
Another gray area of HIV treatment is when a viral load falls between 5,000 and 30,000. This means that HIV is progressing at a moderate pace. On one hand, AIS recommends you begin treatment if your viral load is between 5,000 and 30,000 and you have a T-cell count of less than 500. On the other hand, the DHHS guidelines say that if you have a viral load below 55,000 and more than 350 T-cells, you don't need to start treatment.

VIRAL LOAD OF BETWEEN 30,000 AND 55,000
If your viral load is in the range of 30,000 and 55,000, it means that your HIV is progressing relatively fast. IAS recommends treatment if your viral load is greater than 30,000 regardless of your T-cell count.

VIRAL LOAD ABOVE 55,000
By all measures, a viral load result of greater than 55,000 is considered high and HIV progression is moving very quickly. For example, one study of people with T-cell counts between 201 and 350, who also had viral loads of greater than 55,000, found that the risk of progression to AIDS within

three years was about 64 percent. But don't sweat it, HIV treatment is very effective at reducing the viral load.

Treating HIV now or later?

There's debate about the best time to start HIV treatment. Should treatment be used immediately when people first learn they are infected? Or should treatment be saved until T-cells drop or viral load increases? Currently, there is no right answer; however, trends over time seem to be heading toward a more conservative, wait-as-long-as-possible approach regarding when to start treatment. There are risks and benefits for each option. Months 7 and 9 discuss this topic at more length. For now, however, consider a few of the major themes that have emerged over time.

Pros and cons of when to start treatment
Some considerations to keep in mind

Delaying treatment
- Delaying treatment for as long as possible may help to avoid negative effects on your quality of life. For example, taking HIV medications every day may cause some inconvenience in your life.
- Delaying treatment for as long as possible will help you avoid drug-related side effects—both the long- and short-term side effects. HIV treatment is hardly perfect. In the first month after you start treatment, many people experience intense nausea or stomach upset. In the long run, HIV treatment may adversely affect your heart and may cause body shape changes.
- Delaying treatment also means delaying the chance that HIV treatment will fail once you do start. For example, if your T-cells are high, you might want to wait until your T-cells drop. This way, you can preserve HIV treatment for a time when you may need it most.
- Delaying treatment may help you preserve the maximum number of available and future drug options. The science surrounding HIV treatment gets better every year. Doctors and researchers may discover something next year that they didn't know last year.

Treating sooner
- Treating sooner may help you have an easier time in reducing your viral load and maintaining extremely low levels of the virus over time.

○ Treating sooner may help you prevent permanent damage to your immune system. Research has shown that serious and perhaps irreversible damage occurs when T-cells drop below 200. However, this is not an absolute cutoff point. The closer you get to 200, the more likely you are to experience permanent damage to your immune system.

○ Treating sooner may decrease the chance of your giving the virus to someone else. In a nutshell, if there's less virus in your blood, theoretically you may be less infectious. This is a controversial topic and more research will help infuse the debate with objective data rather than emotion. At present, HIV treatment can't eliminate HIV from your body, so the risk of transmitting the virus to others still exists. Practice safe sex and use clean needles as often as humanly possible.

IN A SENTENCE:

It's important to consider both your T-cell count and your viral load when deciding when to start HIV treatment.

Getting Healthcare

THERE MAY come a time when you need some medical advice. You might only need simple suggestions on health insurance. Perhaps you need some guidance on accessing Social Security benefits. Maybe you need to see a doctor right away. If you find yourself in a bad spot and you want face-to-face counsel by someone who knows the ropes of living with HIV, your best bet is to contact an AIDS service organization.

AIDS organizations can be lifesavers. These organizations specialize in providing services to people with HIV. One of the greatest services they offer is tried-and-true experience in helping people get access to healthcare. All the new HIV drugs don't matter much if you can't get them or can't afford to see a doctor.

A recent survey of people with HIV found that 72 percent had incomes of less than $25,000. Only 32 percent had private health insurance and about 20 percent had no health insurance at all. For many people with HIV, becoming affiliated with a local service organization can be the gateway to getting medicine.

"Everybody has to realize if you go into a service organization, it's incredibly bureaucratic," says Jelka Jonker, a counselor at AIDS Project Los Angeles. She explains the reason for the bureaucracy stems from the funds these organizations get from state and federal agencies. These organizations must fulfill certain requirements to prove to their funders that they are, indeed, providing services to the people who need them most.

"It can be frustrating when you first start out," says Jonker, "but it's not impossible. Once you're in the system, however, you have access to a lot of critical things. It's important to know that from the beginning."

Tim L. offers some advice for initially cracking the AIDS service organization system. "Have patience," he says. "You have to go to each organization to get a specific service. You can't expect one organization to have everything. You can't go in there and demand things. You have to be patient. If you sit there and be patient, you get the things you need quicker. If they say they're busy, say 'I don't mind, I'll just sit here and wait.' And you know what? They will get you in."

Cracking the HIV system may take some time, but there is a payoff. There's plenty of experience and knowledge to be found in these organizations. So if you find yourself with questions or concerns about getting good healthcare—or keeping the healthcare you have—know that help is out there should you need it.

Service organizations can help with health insurance

There are two types of health insurance: group plans and individual plans. A group health plan is health insurance usually offered by an employer or by a union. Sometimes, these plans allow you to insure dependents as well. An individual plan is insurance sold by HMOs or other issuers to individuals. Remember, although health coverage might be offered through an association, a college, or a group of self-employed individuals, it's probably still considered an "individual" health plan.

Like it or not, an HIV diagnosis makes you a "substandard risk," which means you're an expensive person to keep around. Insurance companies don't like paying for your medical expenses. In fact, some insurance companies will use every trick in the book to drop your coverage.

For group plans, some insurance companies pass these extra expenses on to your employer, which can sometimes be a strike against you since you cost more to insure than the average employee. For individual plans, most insurance companies won't even offer you coverage, and if they do, it will be extremely expensive.

A recent report on the availability of coverage for people with "less than perfect health" showed that HIV-positive people were routinely denied

individual coverage. The researchers studied six hypothetical applicants—
each with a different medical problem—and all the applicants were given
the opportunity to apply for coverage, except the one with HIV.

So if you have health insurance currently, it's a wise idea to keep the plan
for as long as possible. One way to do this is by knowing about the Health
Insurance Portability and Accountability Act of 1996, known as HIPAA.
This relatively new law may:

○ increase your ability to get health coverage for yourself and your
dependents if you start a new job
○ lower your chance of losing existing healthcare coverage, whether
you have that coverage through a job, or through individual health
insurance
○ help you maintain continuous health coverage for yourself and your
dependents when you change jobs
○ help you buy health insurance coverage on your own if you lose coverage under an employer's group health plan and have no other
health coverage available

Among its specific protections, HIPAA:

○ limits the use of "pre-existing condition" exclusions
○ prohibits group plans from discriminating by denying you coverage
or charging you extra for coverage based on your—or your family's—
past or present poor health
○ guarantees certain small employers, and certain individuals who
lose job-related coverage, the right to purchase health insurance
○ guarantees, in most cases, that employers or individuals who purchase health insurance can renew the coverage regardless of any
health conditions of individuals covered under the insurance policy

In short, HIPAA may lower your chance of losing existing coverage, ease
your ability to switch health plans and/or help you buy coverage on your
own if you lose your employer's plan and have no other coverage available.
However, HIPAA does not require employers to offer or pay for health coverage, it's no guarantee of health coverage for all workers, and it does not
eliminate all use of preexisting condition exclusions. Also remember that
you need at least eighteen months of previous health insurance coverage—
without a significant break in coverage—to take advantage of HIPAA
protections.

COBRA *may help when you change jobs*

One federal law that may help you make the most of HIPAA protections is the Consolidated Omnibus Budget Reconciliation Act of 1985 (COBRA). COBRA allows you to keep your health insurance for up to thirty-six months if you leave your job. However, you'll need to pay extra for it. If you worked for a small company with less than twenty employees, your employer does not have to offer COBRA.

If you're between jobs, COBRA can help you avoid a significant break in coverage. That, in turn, may allow you to shorten or eliminate a preexisting condition clause under a new plan offered by a new employer. But remember, COBRA can be very tricky and subject to cumbersome rules and regulations. For example, if you miss just one payment, you can lose COBRA coverage.

If you're concerned about health insurance, ask a specialist

The rules and regulations involved with health insurance, HIPAA, and COBRA are extremely complicated. There's fine print everywhere. Generally, AIDS service organizations can provide you with help in navigating the shark-infested health insurance waters. As a first step, you can contact the Centers for Medicare & Medicaid Services at (877) 267-2323 or visit their Web site at http://cms.hhs.gov.

The Medical Information Bureau is watching you

The Medical Information Bureau (MIB) is a little like a credit reporting company, but instead of tracking your credit, the MIB tracks your health. If you have ever applied as an individual for life, health, or disability insurance, your name probably is listed with MIB. This company provides details on more than fifteen million Americans and Canadians to about 750 insurance companies. MIB claims that the service it provides to insurance companies helps to fight fraud on the part of consumers applying for health coverage.

As with credit reporting agencies, most of the information stays on record with MIB for seven years. Although you are supposed to be notified when someone is checking MIB's database for information about you, it doesn't always happen. For nine dollars, you can request a copy of your

MIB file by logging onto the Medical Information Bureau's Web site at http://www.mib.com.

A word of advice: If you have HIV, think very carefully about applying for health or life insurance. Once MIB has a record of you being denied for insurance, you're considered a substandard risk. This means you could have a rough time finding health, life, or disability insurance in the future.

You can get good health insurance, but it takes persistence

If you do get dinged for having HIV, don't despair. There are high-risk insurance programs designed just for people who can't get health insurance because of serious or expensive medical conditions. These programs are exactly like commercial health insurance in that they charge premiums, copayments, and deductibles for a defined benefits package.

Although the premiums can be a little higher than regular insurance plans, the coverage is usually excellent and surprisingly affordable. For many years, I was covered by a high-risk insurance plan in Illinois. To qualify, I had to prove that I was denied coverage—but that was the easy part.

There's paperwork and details, and a lot of waiting around for forms in the mail. But in the end, I found the coverage to be on par with—or better than—most individual or group insurance plans. If you can't get health insurance any other way, these programs are definitely the way to go. A word of advice: Many of these state-sponsored programs have long waiting periods for enrollment, so start the process early—even if it's just calling for information. You can start the process by calling your state's AIDS hotline (see Resources section) and asking for the telephone number for your state's program.

Programs are available to help you get HIV-related drugs

ADAP (pronounced "ay-dap") is how most people refer to the AIDS Drug Assistance Programs. The programs provide HIV and AIDS-related prescription drugs to people living in the United States and Puerto Rico who don't have health insurance or who have inadequate health insurance. The program started in 1987 and was dramatically expanded during the 1990s. Every year, Congress allots a certain amount of money to individual states to spend on these programs and this funding can vary from year to year, depending on national fiscal and political trends.

When Congress gives the money to the states, it mandates that the money be spent to "provide therapeutics to treat HIV disease or prevent the serious deterioration of health arising from HIV diseases in eligible individuals, including measures for the prevention and treatment of opportunistic infections."

From there, individual states determine the criteria that a person must meet in order to qualify for the program in that state. For example, you might qualify for New York's program but not for the program in Texas. The states also decide which specific drugs they will offer. So you might have access to a certain drug if you live in California, but not if you live Florida. Both the criteria that a person must meet to be eligible and the drugs offered by the programs can vary from year to year.

Examples of Eligibility in ADAP

EVERY YEAR the eligibility for ADAP changes. Two examples of the criteria to qualify for ADAP are listed below to give you a sense the requirements.

NORTH CAROLINA
- Your income must be at or below 125 percent of the current federal poverty level (in 2003, the poverty level was $8,980, so your income must be at or below $11,225)
- You must be HIV-positive
- You must be a resident of North Carolina
- You must have no private health insurance or Medicaid
- A limited number of people can be in the program, so there is a waiting list

MICHIGAN
- Your income must be at or below 450 percent of the current federal poverty level (so your income must be at or below $40,410)
- You must be HIV-positive
- You must be a resident of Michigan
- You must first apply for Medicaid and have been recently denied
- You cannot be eligible for Veteran's benefits

Getting started: Use the Resources section in this book to find your state's AIDS hotline. The hotline will provide you with the specific details of your state's ADAP program.

Joining a clinical trial is one way to get medical care

Clinical trials are carefully designed research studies that examine the safety and effectiveness of experimental treatments. Clinical trials test the effectiveness of new drugs, test standard medications in different dosages, and compare different combinations of medications to see which ones are most effective. Some clinical trials simply observe your behavior without adding or changing medications

Some trials investigate and treat HIV in patients, while other treat complications and co-infections that may accompany HIV, such as opportunistic infections, hepatitis C, hepatitis B, and tuberculosis (TB). But like anything else, there are pros and cons to be weighed.

ADVANTAGES OF JOINING A CLINICAL TRIAL
- benefits from the new treatment
- free laboratory tests and results
- access to treatments not available to the public
- free supplies of standard or new drugs
- regular medical examinations
- satisfaction from improving the care of others with HIV

DISADVANTAGES OF JOINING A CLINICAL TRIAL
- taking new drugs that turn out not to be beneficial or to have side effects or negative long-term consequences
- not knowing whether you are receiving the actual therapeutic drug or a placebo
- more frequent visits for care than would otherwise be necessary
- being restricted from using other treatments or participating in other studies because of requirements of the clinical trial

For information about participating in clinical trials or trial availability throughout the US, call the AIDS Treatment Information Service (ATIS) at (800) 874-2572 or call a local AIDS service organization.

Social Security can be a lifeline for people with HIV

Social security benefits come in several forms. Three that are especially important are Medicaid, Social Security Disability Insurance (SSDI), and Supplemental Security Income (SSI).

MEDICAID

Medicaid is a health insurance program offered by the federal government. Its purpose is to help people with especially low incomes, such as children, pregnant women, the elderly, and people with special disabilities such as AIDS. Medicaid will pay for a variety of medical services, including visits to the hospital, visits to the doctor, blood tests, home healthcare, and family planning.

In most cases, childless adults living with HIV qualify for Medicaid only after they qualify for Supplemental Security Income (SSI). To be eligible for SSI, you must be disabled. HIV-positive people without symptoms don't automatically qualify for Medicaid until they have full-blown AIDS. However, some states have a special arrangement with the federal government, allowing these states to extend Medicaid benefits to non-disabled people living with HIV.

SOCIAL SECURITY DISABILITY INSURANCE (SSDI)

Most people qualify for Social Security disability by working, paying Social Security taxes, and in turn, earning "credits" toward eventual benefits. The dollar amount of your benefit depends on how much you earned in the past. Generally, higher earnings mean higher benefits. You can—and should—keep track of your earning history. If you find a discrepancy, have it corrected sooner rather than later.

SUPPLEMENTAL SECURITY INCOME (SSI)

SSI is a program that pays monthly benefits to people with low incomes and limited assets who are sixty-five or older, blind, or disabled. SSI supplements your income up to a certain level. The level varies from one state to another.

There are a lot of complicated rules about what specifically counts as income, so this is one area where an AIDS service organization can really come in handy. If you work, there are even more rules. People on SSI should have limited assets. Generally, your assets should be under $2,000, or for couples, your assets should be under $3,000. But your home, personal belongings, and car don't count (unless it's an expensive one).

Defining "disability" can be tricky

Disability under Social Security is based on your inability to work. You're considered disabled if you can't do the work you did before and can't adjust to other work because of your medical condition. If you have HIV and have

How Does Social Security Evaluate Your Disability?

SOCIAL SECURITY works with an agency in each state, usually called a Disability Determination Service, to evaluate disability claims. It's a step-by-step process involving five questions:

Step 1–*Are you working?*

If you are working *and* your earnings average more than $700 a month, you're generally not considered disabled.

Step 2–*Is your condition "severe"?*

Your condition must interfere with basic work-related activities.

Step 3–*Is your condition found in a list of "disabling impairments?"*

Social security maintains a list of "impairments" that are so severe they automatically mean you're disabled. If your condition isn't on the list, your condition must be equal in severity to an impairment that is on the list. For women and children with HIV, the list includes some unique impairments. Some of the HIV-related conditions are:

○ Pulmonary tuberculosis resistant to treatment
○ **Kaposi's sarcoma (KS)**
○ *Pneumocystis carinii* pneumonia (PCP)
○ Cancer of the cervix
○ Herpes
○ Hodgkin's disease and all lymphomas
○ HIV wasting
○ Syphilis and Neurosyphilis
○ Candidiasis (thrush)

Step 4–*Can you do the work you did previously?*

If your condition is severe–but not of equal severity as the ones on the list– then you must prove that it interferes with your ability to do the work.

Step 5–*Can you do any other type of work?*

Your medical condition, age, education, past work experience, and any transferable skills are considered.

symptoms that severely limit your ability to work—and if you meet the other eligibility factors—the chances are good that you'll qualify for benefits. On the other hand, if you have HIV but no symptoms, it is much harder to qualify for benefits. Social security officials are becoming stricter with these rules.

Document your impairments

You'll need to document all of your impairments. This may include medical records and blood test results. Remember, you'll need to prove that you have HIV *and* any related conditions. This may include repeated infections; fevers; night sweats; enlarged lymph nodes, liver or spleen; lower energy or general weakness; cough; depression and anxiety; headache; nausea and vomiting; and side effects of your HIV meds, and how they affect your daily activities.

Not all doctors are aware of all the kinds of information Social Security needs to document your disability. Ask your doctor or other healthcare provider to track your symptoms in detail over time and to keep a thorough record of fatigue, depression, forgetfulness, dizziness, and other hard-to-document symptoms.

It's also critical to document how you function day-to-day. This is where your health journal can come in handy (for a reminder on setting up your health journal, see Day 7.) Use your health journal to jot down brief notes about how you feel on each day. Record anything that shows that you couldn't do your regular activities. Be specific. Don't forget to include any psychological problems or how it's affected your job, if you are working.

Bring every detail and document when you apply for benefits

You can apply for Social Security and SSI disability benefits by calling or visiting any Social Security office. In addition, AIDS service organizations usually have on hand most of the needed documents you need to get the paperwork going. Before making the trip to a Social Security office or an AIDS service organization, be sure to bring your

- ○ Social Security number
- ○ birth certificate
- ○ copy of most recent W-2 form (tax return if you're self-employed)
- ○ documentation of how your condition affects your daily activities

O   names and addresses of previous doctors and clinics
O   summary of work history
O   blood-test results or lab work

If you're signing up for SSI, you'll need to provide records that show that your income and assets are below the SSI limits. This usually includes bank statements, rental receipts, or car registration.

Social Security officials often have special arrangements with AIDS service organizations to streamline the claims process. In some emergency situations, you might qualify for up to six months of benefits before a final decision on your claim. For more information, call Social Security directly at (800) 772-1213 or call a local AIDS service organization listed in the resource section in the back of this book.

IN A SENTENCE:

> *AIDS organizations help you with healthcare issues, such as getting and keeping health insurance, programs for prescription drugs, and social security.*

learning

Discrimination at Work

LOUIS HOLIDAY wanted to become a police officer for the city of Chattanooga, Tennessee. He was qualified: He passed a written exam and a physical agility test, consisting of running, jumping hurdles, treading an obstacle course, and carrying heavy weights. In fact, a conditional offer of employment was extended to Holiday, if he passed a psychological and physical examination.

During the physical exam, Holiday informed the doctor he was HIV-positive, even though the city doesn't normally test applicants for HIV, or have a policy that requires applicants to test negative for the virus. Subsequently, Holiday was informed that the city's conditional offer of employment was withdrawn because he had not passed the physical examination.

When Holiday asked why, the city responded that it didn't want to "put other employees and the public at risk by hiring you." The city claimed that Holiday's HIV status posed a health and safety threat to others because of the possibility of blood-to-blood contact during police work. After some time, however, the city recanted because there was no evidence that this was a reasonable assumption. Instead, the city claimed Holiday's HIV played absolutely no role in its decision to withdraw the employment offer.

Holiday suspected otherwise. He took the matter to court on the premise that his rights under the law had been violated by refusing to hire him solely because of his HIV status. The court agreed, saying that Holiday "was entitled to be evaluated based on his actual abilities and relevant medical evidence, and to be protected from discrimination founded on fear, ignorance, and misconceptions."

"This ruling makes it clear that medically related employment decisions, whether they are about HIV or any other disability, must be based on facts about the individual, not based solely on opinion," said Matthew Coles, director of the American Civil Liberties Union's AIDS Project. For employers, the message is clear: You cannot discriminate against employees or job applicants just because they have HIV.

If you have HIV, you also have some protections under the law. Even people who don't have the virus are discriminated against because they're regarded as having HIV. They're protected too.

Our founding fathers guaranteed us a few things

First, understand that you've been granted a basic level of "guarantees" by the federal government. These guarantees are based on the concept that all men are created equal and that the creator of all men—some call this God—has given you the right to life, liberty, and the pursuit of happiness. Of course, how the United States federal government interprets these minimum guarantees changes over time.

At one time in the United States, you could be enslaved because you were black. At another time in history, you could be jailed because you were Japanese. More recently, you could be denied a job because you were a woman.

In 1990, people with HIV got a certain set of guarantees from the federal government. These came in the form of the Americans with Disabilities Act, more commonly known as the ADA. If you have HIV, you're legally considered "disabled." It doesn't mean you can't walk or need a wheelchair, it only means that you have a few more physical challenges than the average American.

Before the ADA, the consensus was that people with disabilities should be institutionalized, that they were a lower class and should be kept out of sight. The disability rights movement is similar to the civil rights movements before it. Before 1990, it had been assumed that hardships of people with disabilities, such as unemployment and lack of healthcare, were due to the disability itself, and not the way society reacted to the disability.

After 1990, excluding and segregating people with disabilities was viewed as discrimination.

Basically, if you have HIV and you're a citizen of the United States, you're considered disabled. If you're disabled and a citizen of the United States, you're legally protected from discrimination. Now, it doesn't mean that it can't happen, it only means that you can do something about it.

The first step is recognizing discrimination

Discrimination happens all the time to people with HIV. It even happens to people who are HIV-negative because it's assumed that they have the virus. How do you spot discrimination? Well, the definition changes depending on time and location.

If you live in Massachusetts in 2003, you're protected from HIV discrimination exceptionally well. The problem is that laws are different in each state. Most laws attempt to stop discrimination, but people don't always agree on how to enforce these laws.

Checklist for proving discrimination

IN A court of law, you usually have to prove a few things before you can legally claim you've been discriminated against. Here are a few of the basic things you must prove:

- ○ **Action and Inaction:** you have to prove that someone *did* something *or did not do* something that causes you harm or injury.
- ○ **Harm and Injury:** you have to prove that something bad—on a physical level—has happened to you, or you were denied the opportunity to get something good.
- ○ **Disparate or Unequal Treatment:** You were treated differently or worse than others because you have HIV.
- ○ **Disparate or Unequal Impact:** This basically means that sometimes certain rules are unfair—even when the rules attempt to be fair.
- ○ **Separate Treatment:** This happens when you're treated differently for irrational reasons.

Laws are like tools: they only help if you use them. Sometimes, just sharing your understanding of the law with the right people—at the right time—can solve your problems, and save everyone time, money, and grief. Other times, you may need to take a stand or make people obey the law.

Louis Holiday went to court because he wanted to make the point that people with disabilities ought to be judged on the basis of their abilities; that they should not be judged nor discriminated against based on unfounded fear, prejudice, ignorance, or mythologies; people ought to be judged on the relevant medical evidence and the abilities they have. The court agreed.

The ADA spells out your protections

The ADA gives civil rights protections to people with HIV in a similar way to those provided to people with issues of race, color, sex, national origin, age, and religion. It guarantees equal opportunity for people with disabilities in public accommodations, employment, transportation, and state and local government services. If you have HIV, you're protected by the law. Persons who are discriminated against because they are regarded as being HIV-positive are also protected.

The ADA makes rules for dos and don'ts in employment situations

The ADA prohibits discrimination by all private employers with 15 or more employees. In addition, the ADA prohibits all public entities, regardless of the size of their workforce, from discriminating in employment against qualified individuals with disabilities.

The ADA prohibits discrimination in all employment practices. This includes not only hiring and firing, but job application procedures (including the job interview), job assignment, training, and promotions. It also includes wages, benefits (including health insurance), leave, and all other employment-related activities.

In Real Life:

Examples of *employment discrimination* against people with HIV include:

- an automobile manufacturing company that had a blanket policy of refusing to hire anyone infected with HIV
- an airline that extended an offer to a job applicant and then rescinded the offer when, after the applicant took an HIV test as part of the airline's required medical examination, the applicant tested positive

○ a restaurant that fired a waitress after learning that the waitress had HIV

○ a university that fired a physical education instructor after learning that the instructor's boyfriend had HIV

○ a company that contracted with an insurance company that had a cap on health insurance benefits provided to employees for HIV complications, but not on other health insurance benefits

"Reasonable accommodation" can be a slight moderation

A "reasonable accommodation" is any modification or adjustment to a job, the job application process, or the work environment that will enable a qualified applicant or employee with a disability to perform the essential functions of the job, participate in the application process, or enjoy the benefits and privileges of employment.

Examples include: making existing facilities readily accessible to and usable by employees with disabilities; restructuring a job; modifying work schedules; acquiring or modifying equipment; and reassigning a current employee to a vacant position for which the individual is qualified.

IN REAL LIFE:

Examples of *reasonable accommodation* against people with HIV include:

○ An HIV-positive accountant required two hours off, bimonthly, for visits to his doctor. He was permitted to take longer lunch breaks and to make up the time by working later on those days.

○ An HIV-positive computer programmer suffered bouts of nausea caused by his medication. His employer allowed him to work at home on those days that he found it too difficult to come into the office. His employer provided him with the equipment (computer, modem, fax machine, etc.) necessary for him to work at home.

An employer is not required to make an accommodation if it would impose an undue hardship on the operation of the business. An undue hardship is an action that requires "significant difficulty or expense" in relation to the size of the employer, the resources available, and the nature of the operation. Determination as to whether a particular accommodation poses an undue hardship must be made on a case-by-case basis.

• • •

Customer or co-worker attitudes are not relevant. The potential loss of customers or co-workers because an employee has HIV does not constitute an undue hardship. An employer is not required to provide an employee's first choice of accommodation. The employer is required to provide an effective accommodation that meets the individual's needs.

An employer is only required to accommodate a "known" disability of a qualified applicant or employee. Thus, it is the employee's responsibility to tell the employer that he or she needs a reasonable accommodation. If the employee doesn't want to disclose HIV status, it may be sufficient for the employee to say that he or she has an illness or disability covered by the ADA, that the illness or disability causes certain problems with work, and that the employee wants a reasonable accommodation. However, an employer can require medical documentation of the employee's disability and the limitations resulting from that disability.

Sometimes employers are concerned about the future

Employers cannot choose *not* to hire a qualified person now because they fear the worker will become too ill to work in the future. The hiring decision must be based on how well the individual can perform now. In addition, employers cannot decide to *not* hire qualified people with HIV or AIDS because they are afraid of higher medical insurance costs, workers compensation costs, or absenteeism.

Some employers can consider safety when hiring people with HIV

An employer may consider health and safety when deciding whether to hire an applicant or retain an employee who has HIV only under limited circumstances. The ADA permits employers to establish qualification standards that will exclude individuals who pose a direct threat—i.e., a significant risk of substantial harm—to the health or safety of the individual or of others, if that risk cannot be eliminated or reduced below the level of a "direct threat" by reasonable accommodation.

However, an employer may not simply assume that a threat exists; the employer must establish through objective, medically supportable methods that there is a significant risk that substantial harm could occur in the workplace. By requiring employers to make individualized judgments based on reliable medical or other objective evidence—rather than on generalizations, ignorance, fear, patronizing attitudes, or stereotypes.

The ADA recognizes the need to balance the interests of people with disabilities against the legitimate interests of employers in maintaining a safe workplace. Transmission of HIV will rarely be a legitimate "direct threat" issue.

It is medically established that HIV can only be transmitted by sexual contact with an infected individual, exposure to infected blood or blood products, or perinatally from infected mother to infant during pregnancy, birth, or breastfeeding. HIV cannot be transmitted by casual contact. Thus, there is little possibility that HIV could ever be transmitted in the workplace.

IN REAL LIFE:
Examples of *assumed threat* and HIV include:

○ A superintendent may believe that there is a risk of employing an individual with HIV disease as a schoolteacher. However, there is little or no likelihood of a direct exchange of body fluids between the teacher and her students, and thus, employing this person would not pose a direct threat.

○ A restaurant owner may believe that there is a risk of employing an individual with HIV as a cook, waiter or waitress, or dishwasher, because the employee might transmit the disease through the handling of food. However, HIV and AIDS are specifically not included on the Centers for Disease Control and Prevention list of infectious and communicable diseases that are transmitted through the handling of food. Thus, there is little or no likelihood that employing persons with HIV in food handling positions would pose a risk of transmitting HIV.

○ A fire chief may believe that an HIV-positive firefighter may pose a risk to others when performing mouth-to-mouth resuscitation. However, current medical evidence indicates that HIV cannot be transmitted by the exchange of saliva. Thus, there is little or no likelihood that an HIV-infected firefighter would pose a risk to others.

Having HIV can impair your ability to do the job

Having HIV might impair your ability to perform certain functions of a job, thus causing the individual to pose a direct threat to the health or safety of the individual or others.

In Real Life:
Examples of *direct threat* and HIV include:

○ A worker who operates heavy machinery and who has been suffering from dizzy spells caused by the medication he is taking might pose a direct threat to his or someone else's safety. If no reasonable accommodation is available (e.g., an open position to which the employee could be reassigned), the employer would not violate the ADA by laying off the worker.

○ An airline pilot who is experiencing bouts of dementia would pose a direct threat to the safety of passengers. It would not violate the ADA if the airline prohibited her from flying. As noted above, the direct threat assessment must be an individualized assessment.

Any blanket exclusion—for example, refusing to hire persons with HIV because of the attendant health risks—would probably violate the ADA as a matter of law.

Employers should not ask about HIV

An employer may not ask or require a job applicant to take a medical examination before making a job offer. It cannot make any pre-offer inquiry about a disability or the nature or severity of a disability. However, an employer may ask questions about the ability to perform specific job functions.

After a person starts work, a medical examination or inquiry of an employee must be job-related and consistent with business necessity. Employers may conduct employee medical examinations where there is evidence of a job performance or safety problem, when examinations are required by other Federal laws, when examinations are necessary to determine current "fitness" to perform a particular job, and/or where voluntary examinations are part of employee health programs.

Employers should keep your HIV status confidential

The ADA requires that medical information be kept confidential. This information must be kept apart from general personnel files as a separate, confidential medical record available only under limited conditions.

Employers shouldn't discriminate with health insurance

The ADA prohibits employers from discriminating on the basis of disability in the provision of health insurance to their employees and/or from entering into contracts with health insurance companies that discriminate on the basis of disability.

Insurance distinctions that are not based on disability, however, and that are applied equally to all insured employees, do not discriminate on the basis of disability and do not violate the ADA.

Thus, for example, blanket preexisting condition clauses that exclude from the coverage of a health insurance plan the treatment of all physical conditions that predate an individual's eligibility for benefits are not distinctions based on disability and do not violate the ADA. A preexisting condition clause that excluded only the treatment of HIV-related conditions is a disability-based distinction and would likely violate the ADA.

If you think you've been discriminated against in employment

If you believe that you've been discriminated against, the first step is to try to educate the employer about what the ADA requires. If the issue isn't resolved satisfactorily, you can file a complaint with the nearest Equal Employment Opportunity Commission office within 180 days of when the discrimination occurred.

This office will investigate the complaint and either act to correct the problem or give the employee a "right to sue" letter. The right to sue letter permits the employee to sue the employer directly. The employee may be entitled to the job he or she was denied, back pay, benefits, or other compensatory and punitive damages.

For more information about the ADA's employment requirements, call Equal Employment Opportunity Commission at (800) 669-4000.

ADA prohibits state and local governments from discriminating because of HIV

The ADA applies to all state and local governments, their departments and agencies, and any other instrumentalities or special purpose districts of state or local governments.

IN REAL LIFE:
Examples of *state or local discrimination* and HIV include:

○ A public school system that prohibits an HIV-positive child from attending elementary school.
○ A county hospital that refuses to treat persons with HIV.
○ A state-owned nursing home that refuses to accept patients with HIV. A county recreation center that refuses admission to a summer camp program for a child whose brother has HIV.

If you think that state or city government is discriminating against you or your family

If you believe that you're being discriminated against by a state or local government, first try to educate officials involved about the ADA's requirements. You may also file a complaint with the Department of Justice. Complaints must be filed within 180 days of when the discrimination occurred.

COMPLAINTS SHOULD BE SENT TO:
US Department of Justice
Civil Rights Division
Disability Rights Section
Post Office Box 66738
Washington, D.C. 20035-6738

As a last resort, you can sue the pants off them

You also have the right to bring private ADA lawsuits against state and local governments to seek relief, compensatory damages, and reasonable attorney's fees.

ADA Employment questions
(800) 669-4000

ADA Employment documents
(800) 669-3362

Office of AIDS and Special Health Issues
(301) 443-0104

National AIDS Program Office
(202) 690-5471

Bulletin Board System
(202) 690-5423

IN A SENTENCE:

> *Having HIV might result in discrimination, but you have some protections under the law.*

HALF-YEAR MILESTONE

You are now halfway through your first year with HIV.

○ YOU KNOW THAT ONLY CERTAIN SEXUAL BEHAVIORS CAN TRANSMIT HIV, AND THAT COMMON SEXUALLY TRANSMITTED DISEASES, SUCH AS HERPES AND HPV, CAN IMPACT YOUR HEALTH IN THE LONG TERM.

○ YOU UNDERSTAND THAT ANXIETY, DEPRESSION, AND THOUGHTS OF SUICIDE ARE COMMON AND NORMAL AND OPTIONS ARE AVAILABLE TO YOU FOR TREATING THESE CONDITIONS.

○ YOU'RE AWARE THAT SUBSTANCE ABUSE, ADDICTION, AND COMPULSIVE BEHAVIOR START WITH YOUR GENES, AND TREATING THESE CONDITIONS CAN IMPROVE YOUR ODDS FOR SUCCESSFUL HIV TREATMENT DOWN THE ROAD.

○ YOU KNOW THAT A NUTRITIOUS DIET WITH MORE FRUITS AND VEGETABLES AND REGULAR CARDIO AND STRENGTH TRAINING ARE IMPORTANT WHEN YOU HAVE HIV.

○ YOUR UNDERSTANDING OF HIV, THE IMMUNE SYSTEM, T-CELL COUNTS, AND VIRAL LOADS ARE BECOMING MORE SOPHISTICATED.

O You are aware of organizations that can help you with healthcare issues, prescription drugs, social security, and HIV discrimination issues.

The Game Plan for HIV Treatment

YOU DON'T need to know everything about medicine to make a good decision about HIV treatment. You only need to know things that are *relevant* to you, details that are likely to have meaning for you. Imagine that you need a new car. To purchase a car, you don't need to understand how every nut and bolt works—unless you're a car buff and you enjoy learning the finer points. Choosing an HIV treatment strategy is a similar process.

A treatment strategy is a game plan, a set of beliefs that are important for you. For example, some people only buy American cars out of patriotism, while others buy German cars for better performance. Some people drive a lot, so they need a dependable vehicle, while others want better gas mileage or improved safety features. All of these considerations are part of a car-buying strategy.

For HIV, adopting a treatment strategy is not the same as picking the individual drugs. Your strategy may be to wait as long as possible without HIV treatment. However, if your T-cells are low, you may have fewer choices about your strategy. If your T-cells are extremely low, you may need to launch a "shock and awe" assault on the virus very soon so that your immune system can rebuild itself.

As with all big decisions, don't forget to read the fine print. If you're considering declaring war on the virus, understand what that choice may cost you—now and down the road. HIV treatment may be inconvenient, it may disrupt your life, it may cause short- and long-term side effects, and it may be expensive. On the upside, HIV treatment can save your life, and just may extend your good health indefinitely.

If ever there's a time in your life to be a smart and informed consumer, it is now. If you rush into buying a car and end up with a lemon, well, it's a hassle and you're out a few dollars. If you rush into HIV treatment, the consequences are much greater. Sure, you can switch medications down the road, but your first shot at HIV meds is your best shot.

Before you actually begin the medication, weigh the pros and the cons of your strategy. Discuss your thoughts with your doctor. Listen to his or her opinions as well. Don't hesitate to get a second opinion from another doctor either. Then, make peace with your choices.

Step one: look at the whole picture of your health

According to Anthony Fauci, M.D., people with HIV need to start thinking not just in terms of the virus, but in the totality of their health. "Like any other condition, you're treating the *whole* person. The whole person has many other things going on. You're not just treating a virus anymore."

What Fauci is alluding to is the big picture, all the aspects that make up your life and your health. Some aspects of your life may have little to do with medicine. For example, you might not be emotionally ready to begin HIV treatment. You might be between jobs or concerned about money. For some, substance abuse issues may be more urgent these days. (In fact, you'll benefit more from HIV treatment if you're not using drugs or alcohol.) You might not have health insurance or access to decent medical care.

Then there are medical aspects that may be unrelated to HIV. Many people with HIV also have chronic hepatitis C virus (HCV) or chronic hepatitis B virus (HBV). In some cases, the decision to treat HCV or HBV will likely influence your game plan for HIV. These are all factors that figure into your decision to start—or not start—HIV treatment.

Step two: know your T-cells, your viral load, and where they're headed

If you are getting major symptoms associated with HIV, your game plan is relatively clear: start treatment soon. If you're experiencing minor symptoms or no symptoms, you may fall into the gray zone of HIV treatment. In this zone, there's no yes-or-no answer as to the best time to start treatment. In the gray zone, other factors become more important. They might include hepatitis, other preexisting health conditions, substance abuse, your family or financial situation, and your current emotional state.

Another consideration is the fact that HIV treatment is constantly changing. Years ago, conventional wisdom held that people with HIV should treat the virus at any stage in the hope that the virus would be eradicated from the body. This strategy was called "hit hard, and hit early." It's based on the idea that a patient should take the most potent HIV drugs as early as possible. However, the emergence of new long-term treatment side effects has put into question this strategy, and pharmaceutical companies have recognized the need for development of less toxic viral agents for long-term treatment.

"Hit hard, but wait longer" is the new mantra for treating HIV. This new strategy is based on a large and growing body of research that shows very little benefit for people who start treatment when their T-cells are above 350. For people with T-cell counts between 200 and 350, the decision is a judgment call, one that should take the totality of your health into account. Several recent studies have shown that starting therapy when your T-cell counts are between 200 and 350 might mean fewer problems and a lower cost of care because of the fewer complications. If your T-cells are higher than 350, taking treatment may be worse for your health than taking nothing at all.

On the other hand, T-cells are only half the picture. The other half is your HIV viral load. Your viral load is especially important if your T-cells are between 200 and 350. For example, if you had 290 T-cells and a low viral load (less than 20,000 copies), some doctors may want to start you on treatment while others may not. If you had 290 T-cells and a high viral load (greater than 50,000), most doctors would agree that starting treatment is a good decision.

T-cells and viral loads are complicated enough, but it's important to remember that individual T-cell and viral load results are just a snapshot of a moving target. You should consider where your T-cells and viral load are headed. Are your T-cells declining quickly? Or are they staying stable over time? In the same way, knowing if your viral load is increasing or decreasing over time helps you get a better picture of your health.

"If a month ago you were at 1,000 [T-cells], then two weeks later you were at 700, and today you're at 400, that's quite different than having 400 a month ago and today you're at 420. In the later case, you're obviously not sloping down." says Fauci.

Understand you have the power to control the virus whenever you need it

This is perfectly clear: people with HIV in developed countries are no longer dying of HIV disease—as long as HIV treatment is started correctly. An indisputable body of evidence shows disease and death are dramatically reduced by HIV treatment. In fact, according to Bernard Hirschel, an HIV researcher who recently presented the findings of a key study, the risk of death for people beginning HIV treatment is no greater than the risk of death for people who are HIV-negative. He added that "most treated patients will maintain an undetectable viral load," noting that it's "surprisingly uncommon" that treatment fails to suppress the virus.

The good news doesn't stop there. The benefits of treatment last a long time. HIV treatment is extremely effective at suppressing the virus in the majority of people who are "naïve" to HIV medications ("drug-naïve" doesn't mean that your stupid about drugs, it simply means that you've never taken HIV treatment before).

A recent study has confirmed the durability of HIV treatment. Researchers examined people who were taking HIV meds and found that, if patients achieved an extremely low viral load (less than 50 copies) from treatment, then benefits lasted for at least four years. Of course, it may last much longer, but the drugs haven't been around long enough to say for sure. Most researchers agree that the benefits are likely to last for twenty years or more.

If you take HIV treatment correctly and you achieve a viral load of less than 50 copies, "the chance of treatment failure is extremely low . . . viral suppression on [HIV treatment] is proving extremely durable in those who can tolerate their regimens over long periods." This study confirms other studies that have made a similar finding regarding the durability of HIV meds.

The bottom line is that HIV treatment works—and it works especially well for drug-naïve people. No matter how you slice it, this is good news.

Longevity and good health is now the rule, not the exception

"When you're dealing with a disease in which the primary issue is cataclysmic—such as life or death due to the virus itself—there's very little wiggle room about what you should do, about whether you should treat or not," says Fauci. He explained that once the medical community takes control of a disease and longevity is common for most people with the disease, then "secondary issues" begin to rise in importance.

"With HIV now, we're struggling with feeling very good about taking it from a universally lethal disease to a manageable disease, but now, in some respects, we have a more complex problem," says Fauci. "How do you take it from a manageable disease to picking off many of the peripheral secondary issues that now are starting to cause morbidity and mortality? It's a big challenge."

Recent studies have shown that HIV treatment is associated with increases in heart disease and metabolic abnormalities. According to Fauci, the side effects from HIV treatment that are now emerging are just the tip of the iceberg. "Whenever you have major perturbations from an infection or chronic administration of powerful drugs, it's amazing what you see five, ten, fifteen, and twenty years down the pike," says Fauci. "Believe me, we are going to be seeing things that go well beyond cardiovascular [risks]."

However, it's important to remember that a potential increase in risk for heart disease does not mean that you will get heart disease. According to Bob Munk, a long-time HIV treatment advocate who has also been HIV-positive for twenty years, people considering treatment ought to put things in proper perspective. "I see people who are freaked out that the risk of heart disease may go up 1 percent without putting it in context that the risk of HIV disease progression and death has gone down by 80 percent."

A sound approach for dealing with long-term side effects is to be ready for them, says Fauci. In this way, you're better able to prevent them from happening or reduce the damage if they do happen. "You have to think in terms of the delicate balance between being aggressive enough to suppress the virus and conservative enough not to inappropriately treat a person that doesn't really need to be treated."

"Hit hard, but wait longer" HIV treatment

In the auto industry, every year brings new cars. Most new cars are just the latest models, which have modified from previous versions. Some new cars are brand-new models and a few of the kinks have yet to be discovered, let alone worked out.

In many ways, the individual drugs that make up HIV treatment are like cars. Some of the older drugs have been reformulated and improved. Some are being used in entirely new ways. Even a brand-new class of drugs is now widely available. While a new drug class can generate excitement, the

**IAS-USA RECOMMENDATIONS
FOR WHEN TO START THERAPY**

○ Patients with symptoms of HIV disease should all be treated

○ Patients with no symptoms *and* T-cells less than 200

○ HIV infection without symptoms *and* T-cells in the range of 200 to 350 only if the rate of T-cell decline is more than 100 per year

○ Patients with no symptoms *and* T-cells in the range of 200 to 350 only if viral load is high (greater than 50,000 copies)

	Viral Load		
T-Cell Count	Less than 5,000	5,000 to 30,000	Greater than 30,000
Less than 350	Recommend treatment	Recommend treatment	Recommend treatment
350-500	Consider treatment	Recommend treatment	Recommend treatment
Greater than 500	Defer treatment	Consider treatment	Recommend treatment

long-term side effects of new drugs won't reveal themselves until the drug has been used long-term.

Exactly when to start HIV treatment is both a science and an art. Experts still say the "hit hard" concept—using combinations of potent drugs—is the right way to go. However, in many instances, the "hit early" part of the dogma has been replaced by "but wait longer."

Why the change of heart? One reason is that researchers have learned that an immune system that has been fairly severely damaged by HIV can recover most of its function if the virus is effectively suppressed. Effective suppression is possible with current medications in HIV disease. Another reason is the growing importance of long-term side effects of HIV treatment.

According to the Department of Health and Human Services HIV treatment guidelines, any patient with symptomatic HIV disease should be treated. Likewise, anyone with a T-cell count less than 200, or who has had an AIDS-defining opportunistic infection, should receive HIV treatment.

However, the guidelines are less certain for people with a T-cell count between 200 and 350. Some experts recommend that these people begin treatment, but this decision depends on other factors, including a high viral load.

DHHS RECOMMENDATIONS FOR WHEN TO START THERAPY

○ Patients with symptoms of HIV disease should all be treated.

○ Patients with no symptoms who have less than 350 T-cells *or* viral load over 55,000 should be offered treatment. Consider the risk of disease progression and the patient's willingness to start therapy. Some experts would delay treatment for patients with 200 to 350 T-cells and viral loads under 55,000.

○ Patients with no symptoms, more than 350 T-cells *and* a viral load below 55,000 do not need to start treatment. They should get regular viral load and T-cell tests. However, some experts would treat these patients.

Clinical Category	T-Cell Count	HIV Viral Load	Recommendation
Severe symptoms	Any value	Any value	Treat
No symptoms	Less than 200	Any value	Treat
No symptoms	Between 200 and 350	Any value	Treatment should generally be offered, though controversy exists
No symptoms	Greater than 350	Greater than 55,000	Some experts would recommend therapy, since the three-year risk of developing AIDS in untreated patients is greater than 30 percent; some would defer therapy and monitor T-cells and viral load more frequently
No symptoms	Greater than 350	Less than 55,000	Many experts would defer therapy, since three-year risk of developing AIDS in untreated patients is less than 15 percent

Most experts now agree that people with T-cells above 350 should not receive HIV treatment, unless they have a very high viral load or HIV symptoms, according to the guidelines. Don't forget, these are only guidelines; they are not rules.

Don't let medical jargon or fancy buzzwords intimidate you

One of the things to know about "experts"—especially in medicine—is that they don't always communicate in a way that makes sense to regular folks. However, a good doctor should be able to understand what the experts are saying—and then tell you what it means for you. However, doctors simply don't have lots of time to spend with patients. It's up to you to meet your doctor halfway.

While the specifics of HIV treatment change quickly over time, there are some general considerations that remain constant. Here's an overview of key considerations:

COMBINATION THERAPY

With HIV, the standard of care is to combine three drugs together at the same time. A long time ago, doctors gave patients only two drugs. Now we know that a two-drug combination is not only inadequate, but it reduces your options in the future. Within developed countries, the term *combination therapy* is used to describe a combination of *three* different HIV drugs.

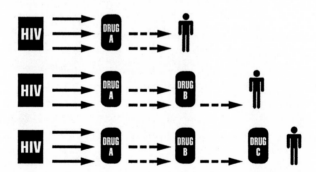

RESISTANCE

Viral resistance is a term often used within the medical community. For all practical purposes, viral resistance is a lot like antibiotic resistance. Another way to look at viral resistance is to imagine that HIV is like a big campfire. Now, imagine the campfire must be extinguished so it doesn't cause a forest fire.

The problem is that you have only three buckets of water. You could throw one bucket on the fire and then wait to see if it works. If the embers that remain smolder for a while and reignite, you've only got two buckets of water left. In the same way, HIV can become resistant to one or many HIV drugs. If treatment doesn't sufficiently snuff out HIV, your viral load may break through all three HIV drugs, making those drugs useless for you in the future.

CAN PEOPLE GIVE DRUG-RESISTANT HIV TO OTHERS?

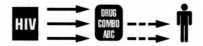

Drug-naïve or *treatment-naïve* are medical terms to describe people who have never taken HIV treatment. Drug-naïve patients generally respond better to HIV treatment than people who have taken treatment sometime in the past. These patients are called *treatment-experienced* or *drug-experienced*.

If someone who's had treatment experience on Combination ABC develops resistance, it means that the virus is now resistant to Drug A, Drug B, and Drug C—and HIV has a pretty good memory. The ABC-resistant form of HIV can stay in someone's body for a long time.

It is possible, but unlikely, that resistant forms of HIV can be transmitted from one person to another. A 2002 report in *The New England Journal of Medicine* showed increasing rates of resistance among people who were recently infected with HIV. Resistance to any HIV drug increased from about 3 percent to 12 percent. The authors point out that if such trends continue, it's not a good sign for the future of HIV treatment. On the other hand, it is surprising that the level of resistance was as low as it was.

Should this make a difference in your HIV treatment strategy? Probably not. Should this make a difference for your behavior if you decide to begin treatment? Most likely yes.

SEQUENCING

Sequencing generally refers to choosing the order of specific HIV drug cocktails as they are prescribed for you over the course of your lifetime. Proper sequencing of individual HIV drugs can help you retain the maximum number of drug options in the future. For example, if you take Combination XYZ, then you may have only two or three options for the future. However, if you take Combination ABC, you might have seven or eight drug options in the future.

The best sequence of drugs, however, might depend on whom you ask. If you ask the pharmaceutical company that manufactures Drug X and Drug Y, the company will claim its products should be taken first. "Anytime I hear someone talking about sequencing, I'm very skeptical," says Bob Munk, an HIV advocate and operator of the AIDS InfoNet. "I have yet to see it really pan out."

Your doctor may have his or her own preferences as well. "Maybe with [some drugs] it does translate into something that's clinically relevant," says Munk. "I think it's hard for a patient to know if this [preference] is a hunch or is it based on science. Or, is this just how my doc likes to do things? A lot of docs—especially the ones who have a lower caseload—just have their favorite regimen. It may be based on good science and it may not."

ADHERENCE

Outside the HIV community, the term *adherence* means *compliance*. It refers to the willingness of the patient to comply with the recommended way to take a specific drug. If, for whatever reason, you miss a dose or you forget to take the drugs as prescribed, researchers would call you *non-adherent*. It's important because if you miss a dose on occasion, your chance of getting viral resistance is much higher.

Of course, things get much more complicated when people take three drugs for several years. One drug should be taken with food, the other with an empty stomach. Some drugs can't be taken at the same time; they need to be taken a few hours apart. It's even possible to misunderstood your doctor or pharmacist and follow the wrong instructions. All of these considerations go into being adherent to medications.

So how do you take three drugs perfectly all the time? Month 10 discusses this topic in more detail. But the short answer is, you don't. It's extremely unlikely for anybody to be 100 percent adherent to their medications over the course of years. The answer to this problem is not always to blame the patient, but also to consider sometimes blaming the drug combination. "We need better treatments that are easier to take," says Munk "We need treatments that are more forgiving. A drug can be more forgiving if there's a margin of safety in case you miss a dose."

ONCE-A-DAY DOSING

Of course, taking HIV meds only once a day is easier than taking them twice day. There are several ways for a drug-naïve person to construct a treatment regimen that's taken only once a day. Those options are likely to increase over time, making once-a-day treatment a standard of care. From a scientific standpoint, studies have shown that patient adherence is better on a once-a-day regimen compared to a twice-a-day regimen.

The downside to rushing too quickly to the once-a-day bandwagon is that it's still not clear if once-a-day regimens are as effective as twice-a-day regimens. Only as more people begin taking once-a-day medications for many years can we be sure. It depends on how much risk you're willing to tolerate versus how much convenience you might gain.

Another downside to once-a-day dosing can be observed if you miss a dose. When you're on twice daily regimens, missing one dose per week means missing treatment for twelve hours or one out of fourteen doses per week (8 percent missed doses). But in a once-a-day regimen, one missed dose equals a missed dose for a whole twenty-four hour period and one missed dose per week equals one out of seven doses or 15 percent missed. This can have large implications when you are trying to keep viral load at undetectable levels and avoid treatment failure.

INTERINDIVIDUAL VARIABILITY

Interindividual variability is a twenty dollar word that means *what's true for the majority may not be true for the individual.* Your genetics, your gender, your diet, your lifestyle, co-infections, and the luck of the draw make you different than, say, the gal down the block. The way your body metabolizes HIV treatment may be different than hers. Even if only one person in a hundred people gets a strange reaction, you may be that hundredth person.

STRUCTURED TREATMENT INTERRUPTIONS

Structured treatment interruptions are an experimental strategy. In this strategy, people start HIV medication, then stop for a short time, and then start again. Don't confuse structured treatment interruptions with *drug holidays*—a phrase people sometimes use when they don't feel like dealing with meds for a few days or a month. Drug holidays are a *really* bad idea. Someday, structured treatment interruptions may lead to a better understanding of the human immune system and HIV. But for now, there are very few practical benefits to this strategy when compared to the risks.

HIV treatment isn't perfect, but it's getting better every year

What would perfect medications be? "They would be 100 percent suppressive of the virus and its replication, they would not have any serious side effects, they would be convenient to take, and their action would be durable.

You could take them for years without worrying about the virus developing resistance," says Munk. "Obviously, we don't have those medications."

Fauci is somewhat more optimistic about the drugs, but reminds physicians to include the concerns of patients. "We have some great drugs, but what about the patient? Do everything in the context of the needs of the patient—the patient's willingness to take a risk, the willingness not to take a risk, or how the patient feels about walking around with a viral load that may not mean anything, or might be slowly and insidiously whittling away at their [T-cells]."

HIV treatment is a work in progress. "That's the good news and the bad news. It's not absolute now," says Fauci. "Right now, the general feeling is that if you've got 400 [T-cells] and 25,000 [copies of HIV] you should wait, that the chances of your getting AIDS in three years is so low that it probably doesn't balance against the toxicities.

"If you had two million copies and 75 [T-cells], I'd grab you by the ears and shake you, 'you really need to be on therapy.' If you had undetectable virus and 800 [T-cells], I'd say you're absolutely crazy for going on therapy. But, in the same breath, I'd say that you need to follow your [T-cells] and follow your viral load."

If you're toying with the idea of going on treatment, Fauci offers four critical tips for people with HIV.

1. **Get a physician whom you trust, who's knowledgeable, who has experience.**
2. **Don't hesitate to get a second opinion.**
3. **Be compulsive about follow-up care.** If you make a decision, remember, this is a dynamic situation that can change. Just don't say, "Well, I've decided I'm not going on therapy" and then disappear for a couple years. Close medical follow-up is very, very important.
4. **Lead a generally healthy life.** When you're dealing with a delicate homeostasis between your body and your body's physiology, you don't want to knock yourself out—get a good night's sleep, don't abuse alcohol, be careful and take time off from work when you're sick, eat a good diet, and exercise.

IN A SENTENCE:

Until we do get perfect medications, HIV treatment will remain as much an art as it is a science.

learning

Meet the Drug Families

EVERY YEAR, the list of HIV drugs grows a little longer. In some cases, pharmaceutical companies have reformulated older, clumsier drugs to make them more useful or practical. In other cases, one drug might be prescribed to boost the potency of another. And remember, just because a drug is new, that does not mean it's better. In fact, there's a higher risk that newer drugs can produce bad side effects, which only show themselves after several years.

With the big picture in mind, here are a few key details about the individual drugs—which when combined—become effective treatment for HIV.

Nucleoside reverse transcriptase inhibitors (nukes)

The nukes are the oldest class of drugs, so doctors know the most about this class. Nukes are generally considered to be the "backbone" of a triple-drug combination. However, which nukes to use first may depend on whom you ask. Some drugs in this class—such as the drug Zerit (stavudine)—are being used less due to the association of metabolic disorders seen in various studies and physicians themselves observing the toxicities to this drug.

Tenofovir (viread) is being used more often because of its safety profile, especially in drug-naïve people. Technically, tenofovir is a nucleotide reverse transcriptase inhibitor. But tenofovir is basically a nuke, according to Munk, who served on an FDA committee to approve the drug. "Don't let anybody tell you that it's a different class. I think [its manufacturer] Gilead would probably love to believe that it's a totally new class of drug. But the reality is that it's not. However, it's a great drug in terms of being forgiving, having very few bad side effects, and in terms of efficacy. It's great. It moves us toward that more perfect regimen."

Nucleoside reverse transcriptase inhibitors (nukes)
Retrovir (zidovudine; AZT)
Epivir (lamivudine; 3TC)
Combivir (AZT *and* 3TC in one pill)
Videx Enteric Coated (didanosine; ddI)
Hivid (zalcitabine; ddC)
Trizivir (abacavir *plus* zidovudine *plus* lamivudine in one pill)
Zerit (stavudine; d4T)
Ziagen (abacavir)
Viread (tenofovir)
Coviracil (emtricitabine)*
Aztec (zidovudine, controlled release)*
*These drugs are in late-stage development

Protease inhibitors (PIs)

Protease inhibitors (PIs) were heralded as a breakthrough in the late 1990s. The addition of PIs to the existing nukes is what tipped the scales toward getting HIV under control. A triple-combination that included a PI is what the general media called the "AIDS cocktail."

PIs are potent. They are extremely effective at reducing HIV. However, the major problems with them are the relatively high number of pills per dose and the long-term side effects. Some of these side effects include body shape changes, elevations in cholesterol, and elevations in triglycerides. A new protease inhibitor called Reyataz (atazanavir) appears to have less negative effect on cholesterol levels, but only time will tell. Additionally, both atazanavir and a new reformulated version of Agenerase (compound 908) have a much lower **pill burden**, which means you take fewer pills per dose. That's good news because PIs in general have a high pill burden.

PROTEASE INHIBITORS (PIs)
Fortovase (saquinavir soft gel capsules)
Norvir (ritonavir)
Crixivan (indinavir)
Viracept (nelfinavir)
Agenerase (amprenavir)
Kaletra (lopinavir *plus* ritonavir)
Reyataz (atazanavir)
Tipranavir*
*These drugs may only be available through clinical trials or special programs

Non-nucleoside reverse transcriptase inhibitors (non-nukes)

As a class of drugs, the non-nukes are older than those of the protease-inhibitor class. The oldest drug is Viramune (nevirapine), which didn't perform well in early tests. It wasn't until Sustiva (efavirenz) came along that the whole class of drugs enjoyed a boost in popularity. Clearly, Sustiva is performing the best overall and continues to prove potent—or more potent—than the PIs without as many bad side effects. However, Sustiva can cause some "mental" side effects such as clouded thinking or unusual dreams.

NON-NUCLEOSIDE REVERSE TRANSCRIPTASE INHIBITORS (NON-NUKES)
Viramune (nevirapine)
Sustiva (efavirenz)
Rescriptor (delavirdine)

Fusion Inhibitors

For drug-naïve people, the importance of this class of drugs is more about the milestone it represents in drug development. The first member of this class is called Fuzeon (enfuvirtide) and it needs to be injected twice a day for as long as you take the drug—and it must also be used in combination with drugs from other classes.

FUSION INHIBITORS
Fuzeon (enfuvirtide)

"More and better" HIV drugs are the direction that HIV treatment is headed, says Anthony Fauci. "There are already indications that there are going to be protease inhibitors that don't have as much metabolic abnormalities, that don't cross-resist with other protease inhibitors. We already have Fuzeon. On the horizon are binding, fusion, and entry inhibitors."

Bob Munk concurs that new classes of drugs are on the horizon. However, he hopes the direction of treatment leans toward "more forgiving" drugs. "What are the long-term side effects of these new classes of drugs?" asks Munk. "No drug ever looks better than the day it gets approved by the FDA. Great, we've got an entry and fusion inhibitor. What does somebody look like after five years on a fusion inhibitor? We won't know until we get there."

IN A SENTENCE:

HIV treatment consists of drugs from various drug families: nucleoside reverse transcriptase inhibitors (nukes), protease inhibitors (PIs), non-nucleoside reverse transcriptase inhibitors (non-nukes), and fusion inhibitors.

Viral Hepatitis

ON THE HIV front, Augustin C. had been doing fine since he got the virus in 1987. For years, his T-cells held steady at around 800, but more recently his T-cells have been inching downward while his viral load has been creeping slowly upward. Right now, he's not worried about HIV, he says. What's on his mind these days is the **hepatitis C virus (HCV)**.

Augustin C. tested positive for HCV nine years ago. Over the years, his doctors have dismissed his chronic HCV as a "wait and see" situation. For better or worse, Augustin C. put HIV and HCV out of his mind. Until this month.

"Physically, I've always been fairly strong," says Augustin C. "But, one day I was driving and suddenly felt a weird pain, almost a throbbing, in my chest. It was on the right side of my chest, kind of below my ribcage. I know it's my liver. I know I'll need to treat the hepatitis soon."

Augustin C. is not in a unique situation. While the true prevalence rates of viral hepatitis are unknown, it's estimated that between 15 and 30 percent of those with HIV also have hepatitis C. Among gay men who have HIV, about 40 percent also have hepatitis B. Until recently, most doctors overlooked viral hepatitis infections, thinking that HIV-positives wouldn't live long enough to encounter problems from hepatitis.

"It has now become clear, however, that this was a grave mistake," writes Mark Nelson, M.D., a physician at a London-based

HIV unit. In a recent report, he speculates that virus-related liver problems account for about half of all visits to London-based HIV clinics these days.

Statistics, however, don't go far in helping Augustin C. He's made an appointment to see his HMO doctor. For the next three weeks, he's waiting and wondering what to do next.

There are things you can do right away

Right off the bat, there are three important things that people—with any combination of HIV, HBV, or HCV—can do to help themselves.

1. **Stop drinking alcohol.** Using any alcohol and some types of drugs is a major assault on the liver. Research on HIV/HCV co-infected patients shows this population is more sensitive to "alcoholic and drug-related" liver disease. Research in HIV/HBV show similar results.
2. **Get a vaccination to prevent hepatitis A.** Hepatitis A is a common and easily transmitted virus that attacks the liver. The majority of people recover from hepatitis A. However, if your liver is already burdened by other viruses or HIV medicine, Hep A is the last thing you need and can cause major problems.
3. **Find out if your body has defense (immunity) against hepatitis B.** If you don't have immunity to hep B, get vaccinated to prevent it. The hep B vaccination tends to work best in people with higher T-cells, so it's better to get vaccinated sooner rather than later.

Managing co-infection with HCV and HIV is complicated

"Obviously, you need to think about other secondary diseases," says Anthony Fauci, M.D. "You have to have a great familiarity not only with the disease itself, but also with the overlapping and confounding issues of treatment." He explained that both HIV and HCV make each other worse. Adding insult to injury is the fact that the drugs used to treat HIV can worsen the situation with HCV—and the drugs used to treat HCV can worsen the situation with HIV.

At one time, researchers had hoped that HIV treatment would bolster the immune system in a way to help with HCV. The results of new research, however, suggest this is not the case. In one study, people with both HIV and HCV received HIV treatment for a year. While T-cells and HIV viral load improved, the HCV viral levels remained unchanged. The researchers concluded that HIV treatment by itself "will not lead to better control of HCV replication."

For HCV and HIV co-infected people, it becomes a question of "which virus is the biggest threat to my health?" Long-standing HCV disease may lead to development of fibrosis, cirrhosis, liver failure, and liver cancer. One study found that the estimated time from HCV infection to cirrhosis in people with HIV patients was over thirteen years. Another study reported that HCV-related fibrosis advances faster in people with HIV.

Years since infection with HCV	HIV-positive people who developed permanent liver damage	HIV-negative people who developed permanent liver damage
16 years	19 percent	2 percent
20 years	35 percent	3 percent
25 years	65 percent	6 percent

Presently, there are no clear guidelines for patients with HIV and HCV, according to John G. Bartlett, M.D., of the Johns Hopkins University School of Medicine. Writing in The *Hopkins HIV Report*, he noted extraordinary results recently with a new anti-HCV protease inhibitor that "may encourage some to delay today's standard therapy." He noted that the drug may have a number of advantages: "It is orally administered, possibly more effective, and probably better tolerated [than current HCV treatment]. This simply points out the rapid pace of development in the HCV field. . . ."

Recently, the National Institutes of Health issued a consensus statement on managing HCV. The following recommendations were made for when and how to treat HCV among the general population.

When to Treat
    The time to treat is when HCV viral load exceeds 50 IU/mL
plus
    liver biopsy shows portal or bridging fibrosis and at least moderate inflammation
plus
        no active injection drug use, alcoholism, neuropsychiatric disorder, or decompensated liver disease. (Anxiety and depression are examples of neuropsychiatric disorders while cirrhosis, a form of scar tissue, is an example of decompensated liver disease).

What to Treat With
Genotype 1: Pegylated interferon *plus* ribavirin for 48 weeks
Genotype 2 or 3: Pegylated interferon *plus* ribavirin
or
standard interferon *plus* ribavirin for 24 weeks

In each case, treatment may be discontinued at twelve weeks if there is not a decrease of at least two logs in HCV viral load. While these guidelines are aimed at the general population, new research has shown that this twelve-week decision is likely to be valid for HIV-positive people. Preliminary research with pegylated interferon plus ribavirin suggest this treatment may have a promising, if limited, role in "clearing" HCV among HIV-HCV co-infected people. However, side effects and adherence should be closely monitored.

"The consensus that I hear," says Bob Munk, a long-time HIV treatment advocate, "is that if your HIV does not require treatment, then go for the hep C treatment in hopes that you can clear it. It obviously leaves you in a better position so your liver can tolerate the HIV therapy."

It's possible your HCV is okay, but your HIV is the problem

There may come a time when it's prudent to treat HIV and *not* treat HCV. In this population, researchers have reported higher rates of liver problems, some of which were severe. They found an increased risk for liver toxicity from HIV drugs in general, but more so with ritonavir, stavudine, and nevirapine.

The researchers concluded that HIV treatment-induced liver toxicity is "very common in patients co-infected with HCV." They added that T-cells below 250 and lower liver enzymes (ALT) were associated with liver toxicity—but not to the degree that caused increased sickness or death, or interruption of HIV therapy.

As with HIV, the details on the interaction between HIV and HCV change rapidly with time. For up-to-date information, visit http://www.hivandhepatitis.com.

• • •

Managing co-infection with chronic hepatitis B and HIV is more complicated

"There are many patients who cannot think about HIV without thinking about the hepatitis [effects] as well," says Anthony Fauci, M.D. "For HBV, the decision to treat is more complicated because some of the drugs used for fighting HBV are the very same drugs used for fighting HIV."

Fauci offered a word of caution. The damage that HBV causes to the liver comes mostly from the immune system. With HIV, the immune system is suppressed—so there's less damage being done to the liver. However, if the immune system regains strength after HIV treatment, there's the possibility of a "secondary immune reactivation" that might cause some liver damage.

Paradoxically, some drugs for HIV are also the frontline drugs for chronic hepatitis B: lamivudine (Epivir or Epivir-HBV), adefovir (Hepsera), and tenofovir (Viread). Early on, doctors discovered that lamivudine was active against HBV. With time and a somewhat lower dose, lamivudine was approved by the Food and Drug Administration to treat chronic hepatitis B.

The problem with lamivudine is that it doesn't work for long. About 90 percent of people co-infected with HIV and HBV will develop HBV resistance within four years. Luckily, both adefovir and tenofovir can effectively block HBV after lamivudine stops working.

Adefovir began its career as an HIV drug. However, at the higher dosage needed for HIV, the drug caused unacceptable rates of kidney damage and the drug was abandoned for HIV. Instead, its manufacturer sought and received FDA approval to sell adefovir—at much lower doses—to treat HBV.

Tenofovir is another HIV drug with substantial activity against HBV. This is not surprising because tenofovir is chemically similar to adefovir. Today, tenofovir is approved by the FDA to treat HIV only and the manufacturer has no plans to pursue tenofovir for the treatment of HBV. However, limited research has shown that both tenofovir and adefovir may be equally active against HBV. Tenofovir is a more attractive option than adefovir for the treatment of HBV in patients co-infected with HIV.

The anti-viral activity of tenofovir, combined with the drug's excellent tolerability in patients with HIV, gives tenofovir an advantage in this population of patients. Combination therapy for HBV infection (i.e., lamivudine and tenofovir)—although not formally evaluated yet—is also attractive from a theoretical perspective.

According to Fauci, the future of HIV and HBV co-infection is being "worked out" very well. "In the era of antiretrovirals therapies, the long-range prognosis for people with HIV, in regard to their HBV, has changed so dramatically that it's essential to pay as much attention to other issues that were always far secondary—among those, hepatitis is one of the most important."

IN A SENTENCE:

> *For people with HIV, co-infection with either HCV or HBV makes treating any of these viruses more complicated.*

learning

Treating Hepatitis

IF YOU have HIV and HCV or HBV, it's important to ask yourself and your healthcare provider two important questions: How damaged is my liver? and What medications will help or hurt my liver even more?

To help assess the state of your liver, you and your provider should carefully monitor blood levels of **aspartate transaminase (AST)**. AST, as it is generally referred to, is an enzyme that gets into the blood after the injury or death of certain cells. Doctors use AST levels to get a sense of what's happening to your liver.

For both HCV and HBV, it's wise to track the levels of those viruses in your blood. Use your health journal to write down the specific numbers so you can see the trend over time (for details on setting up a health journal, see Day 7). However, for the best picture of the health of your liver, your doctor or healthcare provider may need a liver biopsy. Your doctor may advise you to avoid certain drugs or medications that are especially hard on your liver. However, some medications are available specifically to treat HBV or HCV.

Overview of Treatments for HBV and HCV

	HIV	HCV	HBV
standard interferon	Sometimes used in people with HIV disease to control various secondary viral infections	FDA-approved for chronic HCV; limited effectiveness, many side effects	FDA-proved for chronic HBV; limited effectiveness, many side effects
pegylated interferon	Sometimes used in people with HIV disease to control various secondary viral infections	FDA-approved for chronic HCV; improved effectiveness, many side effects	Studies are being conducted to see if "peg" interferon works better than standard interferon
ribavirin	Previous studies have shown no effectiveness for HIV	FDA-approved when combined with interferon	Effectiveness and safety for HBV has not been established
lamivudine	FDA-approved for HIV as part of a three-drug combination	lamivudine is not used for HCV	FDA-approved for the treatment of HBV; limited effeceness
emtricitabine	Currently being studied for HIV; may be widely available soon	emtricitabine is not used for HCV	Currently being studied for HBV and may be widely available soon
adefovir	Higher doses for HIV have unacceptable risks for kidney damage	adefovir is not used for HCV	FDA-approved for the treatment of HBV in non-HIV patients
tenofovir	FDA-approved for HIV as part of a three-drug combination	tenofovir is not used for HCV	Studies show significant effectiveness for HBV

Liver biopsy is the gold standard for assessing liver damage

Liver biopsies really aren't so scary. Sure, people cringe when I admit to having had two liver biopsies—a diagnostic procedure that retrieves a snippet of liver tissue for examination under a microscope. At first, the procedure sounds reasonable, as the results can give you the bottom line on the health of your liver.

What gives people the heebie-jeebies is how doctors actually get the sample. A specialist jabs a long needle into your chest, between your ribs, which pierces your liver. The needle is hollow, so it draws back a thin, long slice of your liver. The needle jab takes only seconds. I didn't feel a thing either time.

In general, liver biopsies are used to check if your liver is scarred (scar tissue is beginning to replace functioning liver cells), if inflammation (cellular infiltration and swelling) is present, or if necrosis (dead liver cells) are present. When the liver becomes permanently injured, it's called cirrhosis.

My first biopsy was performed at Cedar's Sinai Medical Center in Los Angeles, California. The whole procedure was somewhat like having a tooth removed. I showed up on a Friday morning, received a mild sedative, the doctor held what looked like a staple gun to my chest, and it was over in an instant. I rested over the weekend, had some mild soreness, but I was fine by Monday.

My second biopsy was part of a clinical trial at the National Institutes of Health Clinical Center in Bethesda, Maryland. It was a far more complicated ordeal. I flew to the NIH, and checked into the hospital a day before the procedure. Three or four different doctors and nurses explained—in detail—the risks and benefits of the procedure, which again was painless (but still creepy on a conceptual level).

Moments after the procedure, I asked the NIH surgeon if I could see the liver sample. It looked a little like a worm. I then asked the surgeon if I could keep a small piece as a souvenir. After all, I figured it was mine to begin with.

The surgeon chuckled and replied, "Well, this is really valuable. Every bit of this is going to be examined. There's a lot to be learned from this sample." I figured my request *was* a little weird. I stayed at the hospital for another two days and returned home.

It's possible to get a liver transplant— even if you have HIV

AIDS activist and acclaimed writer Larry Kramer got a new liver recently. Kramer is the founder of an HIV activist group called ACT UP. Founded in 1987, this grassroots coalition made national headlines during the 1990s with well-orchestrated and widely publicized demonstrations designed to influence business and government about AIDS policy.

At sixty-six years of age, and after a widely publicized plea for a liver transplant, Kramer got his wish. These days, he's also got a new soapbox: Cutting the red tape that's required with organ transplant policy in the United States, most notably for people with HIV. Traditionally, people with HIV are excluded from receiving organ transplants.

"In Kramer's case, his HIV has been relatively well controlled without [HIV treatment]. However, like many HIV patients with viral hepatitis, his liver disease continued to progress in spite of anti-hepatitis medications," says John Fung, M.D., chief of the division of transplant surgery at the University of Pittsburgh School of Medicine (UPMC). "For the most part, results have been good and most of our patients can expect to do well after transplantation."

UPMC is one of ten centers participating in a National Institutes of Health-funded study to determine the safety and effectiveness of liver and kidney transplantation in patients with HIV. The results of this study may be useful to the entire transplant and infectious disease community as physicians and surgeons attempt to define the best care for people who are co-infected with HIV and viral hepatitis.

IN A SENTENCE:

If you have HIV and are co-infected with HCV or HBV, your treatment strategy should consider both infections and the health of your liver, which can be assessed by blood tests or a liver biopsy.

Long-Term Effects of Treatment

IF YOU were buying a car, you'd want to know how the car model performs for other people. You'd ask friends, acquaintances, or co-workers about they're experiences. Surprisingly, some people researching HIV treatment go to greater lengths to find the right car than they do to choose the right treatment.

Before you commit to a three-drug combination for HIV, you should be aware of some of the long-term side effects these drugs might cause. Of course, you'd want to know how *likely* some of these side effects are to happen. On the other hand, even if a side effect is unlikely, you should also consider what the side effect could mean for you should it occur down the road.

Clearly, there's been increasing reports of metabolic effects. They include:

- ○ insulin resistance
- ○ glucose intolerance
- ○ dyslipidemia (high levels of fat levels in the blood)
- ○ changes in body fat distribution
- ○ lactic acidemia (buildup of lactic acid)
- ○ osteopenia (bone disease)

There is a lot of debate right now among patients, doctors, and researchers about what exactly is at the root of these abnormalities. In fact, it's not even perfectly clear that these abnormalities come directly from the HIV meds.

What is clear is that these long-term side effects can eat away at your quality of life. The side effects may even put you at a higher risk for heart disease. Although there are no approved therapies for body fat changes, some doctors and patients have begun to use unproven therapies, which sometimes help and sometimes hurt patients.

The International AIDS Society—USA has prepared a document that discusses many of the leading theories, risk factors, and potential treatments that have surfaced in recent years. This document summarizes the various debates taking place about these abnormalities. Its purpose is to guide physicians and patients in making better decisions, to help prevent new conditions from occurring in the future, and to minimize long-term risks. What is clear from the document is that long-term HIV treatment requires diligent monitoring and, in some cases, preemptive treatments.

Insulin resistance and blood sugar abnormalities can occur with HIV treatment

Before HIV treatment, insulin resistance and blood sugar abnormalities were uncommon in people with the virus. For many years, doctors thought these conditions were primarily caused by meds other than the HIV meds. These days, however, the prime culprits seem to be the HIV meds themselves.

Insulin is a hormone produced by the pancreas that does many things, but one of its most important actions is to help cells in the body absorb a special type of sugar called **glucose**. Insulin resistance is a reduced sensitivity in the tissues of the body to the action of insulin, which is to bring glucose into those tissues to be used as a source of energy. Insulin resistance causes the level of insulin in the blood to become dangerously high, and a condition called **diabetes mellitus** develops. In general, insulin resistance is linked to increased risk for heart disease, blood abnormalities, fat metabolism, and blood pressure problems.

Doctors believe that HIV meds might impair the cell's ability to absorb glucose. In fact, about 40 percent of people who take a protease inhibitor (PI) will have abnormal glucose levels due to insulin resistance. Only time will tell if all PIs will lead to such conditions; however, one specific PI called indinavir (Crixivan) is more strongly linked to the condition.

If you're already predisposed to abnormalities related to insulin or glucose, taking a PI might make things worse. For people with these conditions, doctors recommend that fasting glucose levels be checked before and during HIV treatment.

If problems do start to happen, some options are to substitute the PI with one of the following drugs, which have been shown to be a little better in terms of insulin resistance:

○ efavirenz (Sustiva)
○ abacavir (Ziagen)
○ nevirapine (Viramune)

Of course, a healthy diet and regular exercise are recommended for all people with HIV, but for people with glucose abnormalities, this recommendation is particularly critical to prevent worsening of diabetes mellitus.

Abnormal levels of fat in your blood can occur with protease inhibitors

In HIV lingo, the term *lipodystrophy* is often used to describe a number of specific conditions. The word *lipid* means *fat*. The word *dystrophy* means *shrinking*. So the term *lipodystrophy* is accurate for describing the shrinkage of fat in certain areas of you body, but it's technically inaccurate when used to describe the accumulation of fat in other areas. Terms that are more accurate are *lipid abnormalities* or *body shape changes*.

There are different types of lipids in your blood, but cholesterol and triglycerides are especially important. There are two types of cholesterol: high-density lipoprotein (HDL) and low-density lipoprotein (LDL). HDL is the "good" cholesterol, while LDL is the "bad" cholesterol. One way to remember the difference is associate the *H* in HDL with "happy" and the *L* in LDL with "lousy." Triglycerides are a special type of fat known as fatty acids. In general, high levels of triglycerides are a bad thing.

○ **HDL**—high-density lipoprotein ("happy" cholesterol)
○ **LDL**—low-density lipoprotein ("lousy" cholesterol)
○ **Triglycerides**—fatty acids (less is better)

• • •

Long before HIV treatments were instituted, lipid abnormalities were seen in people with the virus. Usually these people had lower than normal levels of lipids in the blood. The constant battle between the immune system and the virus requires plenty of fuel, and lipids are part of that fuel.

Protease inhibitors (PIs) can cause significant increases in LDL and triglycerides. Newer PIs may have less of an effect on LDL or triglycerides, but also may be less effective. One PI in particular, ritonivir (Norvir), seems to be the worst in terms of elevating LDL and triglycerides.

Doctors really aren't sure why PIs cause these abnormalities. They suspect that these abnormalities contribute to an increased risk for heart disease, but many other factors may play a role as well. On the other hand, nucleoside reverse transcriptase inhibitors (nukes) and non-nucleoside reverse transcriptase inhibitors (non-nukes) don't appear to cause these abnormalities as much.

If you already have higher than normal LDL or triglycerides, or you have a preexisting heart condition—or even if someone in your family does—an HIV treatment regimen containing a PI is probably not a good idea. If you're drug-naïve, constructing a three-drug combination without a PI is easy to do.

Should you begin HIV treatment and encounter elevations in LDL or triglycerides, don't worry. You have many options for fixing the problem. The first option is lifestyle changes that include reduced fat intake, weight loss, reduced alcohol intake, and exercise. Recent data supports using the Mediterranean diet to combat these problems (see Month 5 for more details on this). You can also talk to your doctor about trying "lipid lowering" drugs.

Body shape changes can occur in people taking HIV treatment

For some time, doctors thought PIs were to blame for the rising prevalence of body shape changes in people taking HIV treatment. Now they know that nucleoside reverse transcriptase inhibitors (nukes) and non-nucleoside reverse transcriptase inhibitors (non-nukes) also play a role in this condition. Recent large studies, so to speak, suggest that body fat abnormalities occur in almost half of people taking HIV meds.

Body shape changes can happen in different parts of the body. *Lipo-dystrophy*—the shrinkage of fat—may occur in the face and in the legs, arms, and buttocks. Accumulation of fat—called **lipohypertrophy**—may also occur behind the neck, deep within the belly, and in the breasts.

FAT LOSS MAY OCCUR . . .

IN THE FACE

Fat loss in the face can cause sunken cheeks and hollow temples (the space between the eyes and the ears). People with fat loss in the face often fear that people can tell that they have HIV.

IN THE LEGS, ARMS, BUTTOCKS

Thinning of the arms and legs can make people look more muscular. Veins may become more noticeable. Loss of fat in the buttocks may cause them to become flatter than normal.

FAT MAY BUILD UP . . .

BEHIND THE NECK

Lumpy, fatty tissue behind the neck is sometimes called a "buffalo hump."

DEEP WITHIN THE BELLY

The fat makes the belly feel hard, not soft and squeezable like normal belly fat that sits just under the skin.

IN THE BREASTS

Enlarged breasts can occur in both men and women (but it's more common in women).

Again, doctors aren't exactly sure why this happens or how to treat the problems. In most cases, doctors will suggest lifestyle changes such as diet and exercise (both cardio and strength training). In some cases, doctors will switch or substitute individual HIV medications, but this hasn't proved to be consistently helpful. The next section describes in more detail some of the treatments doctors and patients are using to treat or prevent body shape changes.

IN A SENTENCE:

The long-term side effects of HIV treatment can include a number of metabolic abnormalities.

learning

Strategies to Combat Body Shape Changes

IMAGINE HAVING the word "AIDS" tattooed on your forehead. That's how some people with HIV feel when they start to experience body shape changes, especially when they occur in the face. Like it or not, in the gay community, sunken cheeks convey a message: *infectious*. That's a message most people don't want to send.

If you're considering HIV treatment—or have already started on treatment—consider how long-term side effects might affect you. Body shape changes are so troubling for some people that they make a deliberate decision to stop HIV treatment. Other times, people don't consciously think about how the changes are affecting them. They simply start forgetting to take their meds as prescribed.

Whether you're on HIV treatment or not, it's good to know that there are strategies and treatments in the works to combat these body shape changes. Most are still experimental, but this is likely to change with time.

According to the International AIDS Society (IAS), there's no consensus now about whether it's appropriate to treat body shape changes. Regional fat accumulation may cause headaches, difficulty breathing, and interference with exercise and sleep. Obvious fat loss in the face, limbs, and buttocks can be distressing, but they're not life-threatening.

"It was one of my first big fears," say Paul T., who tested positive recently. "Sunken cheeks are the worst aspect of being HIV, for me, because it gives away your HIV status to people. I'm probably more aware of the changes than the average person. Still, in the gay community, everybody knows what sunken cheeks mean."

Treatment for body changes are in works

According to the IAS, the current options and strategies for minimizing or preventing body shape changes include:

Modification of HIV treatment. Studies have not shown much success with stopping a protease inhibitor to reverse buildup of fat deep within the belly, called intra-abdominal fat. In fact, studies have shown that replacing a nuke called stavudine (Zerit) with either abacavir (Ziagen) or AZT (Retrovir) has produced "statistically significant but clinically modest" increases in the amount of fat on extremities such as legs and arms.

Exercise. Both aerobic and resistance exercise have considerable potential as non-chemical interventions for intra-abdominal fat buildup. Moderate exercise is well tolerated in people with HIV and does not increase viral load.

Diet. There are no data to support the role of a specialized diet for people with body shape changes—unless other metabolic abnormalities or weight loss is also a consideration. However, it is prudent to reduce intake of saturated fat, simple carbohydrates, and alcohol, according to the IAS.

Testosterone. Studies have shown that decreased levels of testosterone, a naturally occurring male hormone, are linked to intra-abdominal fat and insulin resistance among men with HIV. Testosterone can cause gain in lean body mass, increased sex drive, and possibly aggressive behavior. Many men with HIV often have low testosterone levels.

Human growth hormone (HGH). HGH is a hormone that enhances tissue growth by stimulating protein formation. A genetically engineered form of HGH, called Serostim, has been approved by Food and Drug Administration as a treatment for AIDS wasting. According to the IAS, HGH has resulted in both "subjective and objective improvements in body composition." However, the benefits stop when the drug is stopped.

• • •

Human growth hormone may work for some body shape changes—but at a price

"I've seen whole lives completely changed because of Serostim," says John Tapia, owner of Injectable Therapy Services in Burbank, California, a boutique pharmacy specializing in HIV and hepatitis treatments. Tapia has been involved in the pharmacy business for over fifteen years. "I've seen people who started off as sickly and scrawny and then suddenly they have a dramatic turnaround. From what I see, it works."

It may work—and a growing body of research shows it does have benefits—but the benefits come at a very high price. One month's supply of Serostim costs about $7,000. Most health insurance plans and some drug assistance programs cover the cost of the medication—but only if you fit the criteria for AIDS wasting.

AIDS wasting is a metabolic disorder that causes the body to consume vital muscle tissue, body organs, blood cells, and lymphatic fluids (lean body mass) for energy instead of primarily relying on the body's stored fat. Before they qualify as "wasting," people with AIDS typically experience a loss of 5 to 10 percent or more of lean body mass.

Since the introduction of the new HIV treatments, the prevalence of wasting has decreased by 77 percent, which mirrors the decreases in full-blown AIDS. However, some people with HIV are using Serostim to counter body shape changes.

"I've been doing Serostim since the day it came out," says Tim G., who was first diagnosed with HIV in 1983. "I don't get worried about [body shape changes] much anymore because of Serostim." He explained that he uses low doses of Serostim along with low doses of an anabolic steroid called Anadrol. He says these drugs are "critical" to preventing body shape changes, at least for him.

Unfortunately, a thriving black market has emerged around the hormone. After reports of over-prescribing by doctors, counterfeiting, and illicit street sales, health officials have begun tightening controls and restrictions for HGH. Some state drug assistance programs do not cover HGH, while others are considering eliminating it from their formularies.

"Years ago, when people got wasting, they would lose the will to live," says Tapia. "Then, Serostim, testosterone, and anabolic steroids completely changed the scene. Today, it's much more about aesthetics, because these [treatments] don't stop HIV. However, they do help control buffalo humps and improve lean muscle mass."

"When a person looks healthy and feels good about themselves, they *are* healthier," says Tapia. "It becomes an issue of one's value to society, if a person feels like they look better, they can socialize and be productive. It's a little like [some kinds of] dental work, which is ultimately an aesthetic issue as well. Society treats you better, it may help you get a better job and make more money down the road.

"Because of the fraud, doctors are more reluctant to prescribe Sersostim—even if it will help the patient," says Tapia. "Doctors don't want to send a red flag for fraud, so they don't want to prescribe. It's becoming a huge dilemma."

IN A SENTENCE:

> *There are investigational treatments and strategies that may help control body shape changes.*

living

Taking Pills Every Day

WE ALL know how the story goes: You finally join that gym down the street. Or, maybe, you finally purchase everything you need for that new diet. This time, you're going to do it. This time, you're going to get the body you've wanted, lose that extra weight, or finally break that nasty habit.

Maybe a week passes and by all measures, you're on target and feeling great about yourself. Then something happens. Your car breaks down. Your boss reprimands you. Your landlord raises the rent. Suddenly, your well-intended self-improvement plans get put on hold or just fall by the wayside.

Research on human behavior shows that radical behavior changes can rarely be sustained over time. Of course, you *can* change your behavior for a while, but you can't stick with it over time. Therefore, you "cheat" and then you feel guilty, which usually leads to even more problematic behaviors.

We are human beings, not machines. We're imperfect, emotional, and generally prefer pleasure to pain. Sticking to an HIV treatment—as prescribed—is not that different from sticking to a diet or an exercise plan. You may know *what* to do, *why* it's important, and *how* to do it, but actually *doing it* over the long term doesn't always pan out.

Obviously, saying yes to cheesecake or opting to watch a TV show over going to the gym have entirely different outcomes than, say, missing a dose or two of your HIV meds. You don't need a doctor, scientist, or counselor to point a finger at you and say, "Take these pills, or else." Generally, people are skilled at feeling "bad" about themselves without the help of professionals.

The motivation to take your HIV meds every day in the right way *must* come from within you. You are the master of your health, life, and future. You have a choice: either take the pills or don't. But remember, every choice you make has consequences for you and for others. Here are a few considerations should you choose to begin HIV treatment.

What exactly does it mean to be adherent?

Doctors define *adherence* as the "extent to which a patient's behavior corresponds with medical advice." This can include whether you keep your appointments, following up if the doctor refers you to another doctor or specialist, following your doctor's advice about health-related things in general, and taking medications according to the prescribed dosage, frequency, timing, and food requirements. The term *non-adherence* means "not" doing these things. From here on, let's just focus on adherence to HIV medications.

By now, you already know that better adherence means better response to the meds. However, let's take a closer look at what this means in real life. First you need to understand what *resistant virus* means. HIV becomes *resistant* when it learns how to *resist* one more HIV drugs. When this happens, the virus no longer responds to treatment—and that's bad.

Research shows that taking your meds less than 50 percent of the time does not lead to resistant virus. That's because the levels of the drug are so low, there's very little pressure on the virus to change. So what happens is the virus continues to multiply and gobble up your T-cells, unfazed by this half-hearted effort to stop it.

On the other hand, if you take your meds more than 95 percent of the time, resistant virus also does not develop. The reason for this is because the virus is basically snuffed out so completely that it can't develop resistance because there's essentially no virus around to become resistant (remember the analogy of the campfire in Month 7). No virus, no resistance.

The big problem comes into play when people are between 70 and 95 percent adherent to their meds. In this range, there are enough of the drugs in your body to really begin to put pressure on the virus. If there's not enough pressure to snuff out the virus entirely, some of it will survive. The virus that survives is resistant and it's especially nasty because it will forever know how to get around the drugs you take. Eventually, this resistant virus will grow and replace the original virus (called "wild type virus").

The lesson: you need to be more than 95 percent adherent to keep the virus at bay for the long run. But what does this mean in your everyday life? Let's look at the actual numbers:

ONCE-A-DAY REGIMEN
Goal: 95 percent adherence

This means you could miss 1.5 doses a month (30 days) and still be okay. Since you have to do better than 95 percent, let's round it up and say you could miss one dose. This means you could miss a dose once a month and not develop resistance. If you were to miss two doses per month, you'd be at around 93 percent adherent—not good enough. Missing three doses a month, you would be about 90 percent adherent. Remember, anything less than 95 percent puts you at high risk for developing resistant virus.

TWICE-A-DAY REGIMEN
Goal: 95 percent adherence

A twice a day regimen is a little more forgiving because you could miss three doses a month and probably be okay. But remember, that's three *doses* not three *days*. If you think in terms of days, you could miss one and a half days and still be okay. But don't fool yourself, missing three doses in a row is worse than missing one dose a day over the span of weeks. It doesn't mean you can take a weekend off from you meds.

Get to know yourself before you begin treatment

You're probably thinking: "No problem, I could easily take my meds every day," with the caveat that you have a "spare day" in case you forget. Well, let's put your thoughts into action. Here's a simple at-home test to assess your own level of adherence:

1. Purchase a thirty-day supply of once-a-day vitamins. It doesn't matter what kind of vitamins, anything that fits your budget or preference. However, it's important that there be exactly thirty pills.
2. Get a calendar and count out exactly thirty days. Take note of your beginning date and your end date.

3. Write your "beginning date" and your "end date" directly on the bottle of vitamins. Now begin taking one vitamin once a day.

4. In one month from now, when you reach the "end day," check the bottle to see how many vitamins are left over.

5. Now, score yourself:

   ○ **one pill** remaining: Congratulations, you're doing better than 95 percent.

   ○ **two pills** remaining: This means you're scoring at about 93 percent, which is pretty good.

   ○ **three pills** remaining: Here you're right at 90 percent adherent. You're on the right track. Think about why you missed those three doses and consider how you can do better.

   ○ **more than three pills**: Anything more than three pills leftover means you're scoring at less than 90 percent. Unfortunately, with HIV treatment you'll either need to earn an "A" or not take the test at all.

Obviously, the results of this simple test should not make or break your decision to begin HIV treatment. But it will help you get a sense of what it takes to be better than 95 percent adherent in the real world. If you're scoring at less than 90 percent, think seriously about what's going on in your life that's preventing you from taking the pills. If you managed to get through the month and missed one dose or less, adherence is unlikely to be a problem for you.

IN A SENTENCE:

> *A simple test will help you understand what it means to be better than 95 percent adherent to your HIV medications.*

learning

Managing Short-Term Side Effects

I CLEARLY recall swallowing the first pills of my three-drug combination. I remember thinking they seemed like an awful lot of pills to take at one time. So I arranged them on the table in front of me and attempted to spell the word *help* in pills. There weren't quite enough.

With a glass of water, they went down easily enough. An hour went by and I felt nothing. A few more hours went by and still, I didn't feel a thing. Then came time for my second dose, and again, no problems. Nothing at all. I thought, this is going to be a breeze—for about one week. Then it hit me: a wave of nausea washed over me while on the bus headed to work. The nausea persisted. I remember walking past a Starbucks and the smell gave me the dry heaves.

For about two more weeks, my mouth tasted like I was suck-ing on a dirty penny. The whites of my eyes didn't quite seem white. I felt toxic. I dreaded "pill time" because I knew it trans-lated to several hours of queasiness, hardly a motivator for me.

Finally, I couldn't take it any longer. I called my doctor and said "uncle." I give up. I couldn't imagine feeling like this for-ever. His response? "Well, your T-cells doubled and your viral load is undetectable." With that, everything changed.

With time, the side effects subsided almost completely. With more time, my T-cells tripled and quadrupled. And I haven't seen a viral load above 40 copies since 1996.

Expect some degree of short-term side effects when you first start HIV treatment. Sure, you may be lucky and sneak by without any side effects at all. On the other hand, you may be that one-in-one-hundred person that winds up with a medical rarity. The key is knowing what's normal and what's not. Nausea and diarrhea are common events and will go away with time. Rash and fever, however, can be red flags for more serious situations. It's a good idea to write down any symptoms in your health journal so you can describe them in detail to your doctor and remember what drugs may be causing side effects (for a reminder on how to set up a health journal, see Day 7).

If you begin to experience intolerable side effects, be aggressive with your doctor about communicating your symptoms. Remember, only in rare cases are side effects serious enough to require medical attention. Above all, don't just *not* take your meds because you're going to a party later or because you just don't feel like it. Know that your side effects will subside with time. Down the road, you will get the rewards of better health and a longer life.

Side effects vary greatly from person to person

"Side effects? Nope, I didn't have any, thank God," says Precious J., a treatment advocate for Women Alive, an AIDS service organization in Los Angeles, California. "But it was difficult taking all those pills. I was taking about twenty pills a day. That was hard for me. I learned to get though it."

For Tim L., the story couldn't be any more different. "As the new meds came out, I tried each one of them because I had so many side effects. I didn't last more than twenty days on any of them," says Tim L. "With AZT, I had so much fatigue that I'd open my front door and fall down on the ground, asleep, with the keys still in the door."

"I finally tried Viracept with other meds," says Tim L. "That combination seemed to work. The only side effect at first was diarrhea, but I got that under control with [an anti-diarrhea drug called Lomotil]. Once I adjusted to it, I could maintain things without too many problems. Ninety percent of the time, the diarrhea is under control. Once in awhile I'll get diarrhea, so I'll take more Lomotil. I had some nausea at first. I still have gas, but it's one of those things you learn to live with."

Don't worry about all the drug side effects—just the most common and most severe

First thing, before you take your meds, ask your doctor:

○ What are the *most common* side effects of *all* your meds?
○ What are the *most severe* side effects for *all* your meds?

Remember, you'll be taking at least three different drugs and each one has potentially dozens of side effects. It's probably a waste of time to learn about every side effect for every drug. Instead, focus on the *most common* and the *most severe* ones.

Remember, *interindividual variability* means that what's true for the majority may not be true for the individual. Your genetics, your gender, your diet, your lifestyle, co-infections, and just plain luck make you different from the next person. The way your body metabolizes HIV treatment may be different from how somebody else's body might react.

Studies show that women sometimes experience different, more frequent, and more severe side effects than men. This may be due to the fact that women generally weigh less than men do, but they're usually required to take the same amount of drug. Another possible reason might be hormonal differences between genders.

Many people have an adjustment period when starting HIV treatment. This lasts about four to six weeks while your body adapts to the new drug. During this time, you may have headaches, nausea, muscle pain, or occasional dizziness. These kinds of side effects usually lessen or disappear with time. Don't forget that some side effects may actually be due to anxiety, depression, or stress. Keep your emotions and thoughts in check during the adjustment period.

Consider making the adjustment period easier by taking some time off work or lightening your schedule. See if someone can help around the house or help with children.

Here are some common side effects you'll likely experience and a few ways to manage them:

HEADACHE

Headache is a very common side effect of HIV meds. Expect headaches during the adjustment period. Most times, headaches can be eased by over-the-counter medications like aspirin, acetaminophen, ibuprofen, or naproxen sodium. But check with your doctor beforehand to make sure there are no interactions between these drugs and your HIV meds.

For instant relief from a throbbing head, try resting in a quiet, dark room with your eyes closed. Place a cold washcloth over your eyes. Massage the base of your skull with your thumbs and massage both temples gently, or try a hot bath.

Anticipate when the pain will strike. Avoid or limit foods known to trigger headaches, especially caffeine (from coffee, tea, soft drinks, or some medications), chocolate, food additives (like monosodium glutamate, or MSG), nuts, onions, hard cheese, and vinegar.

NAUSEA AND VOMITING

Nausea and the urge to vomit are absolutely awful feelings. Understand that this side effect is common and will eventually subside. Persistent vomiting, however, can lead to serious medical problems, such as dehydration, chemical imbalances, or damage to your throat. Call your doctor if you vomit repeatedly throughout the day or if vomiting persists or interferes with your ability to keep down your meds.

The BRAT diet—**b**ananas, **r**ice, **a**pplesauce, and **t**oast—can help with nausea and diarrhea. Try some peppermint, chamomile, or ginger tea—they can calm the stomach.

Sip cold carbonated drinks like ginger-ale or 7-Up. Avoid hot, spicy, strong-smelling, and greasy foods. If vomiting occurs, replenish fluids with broth, apple juice, Jell-O, popsicles, or Gatorade.

If nausea or vomiting still persists, don't hesitate to ask your doctor for anti-nausea medications such as compazine or Marinol—they can help immensely.

DIARRHEA

Diarrhea is extremely annoying, extremely common, but also very manageable. If you experience persistent diarrhea, first replenish lost liquids by drinking plenty of fluids, like Gatorade, ginger ale, chicken or beef broth, herb tea, or just plain water. The BRAT diet can help somewhat with this side effect.

Try anti-diarrhea medications like Lomotil, Kaopectate, Immodium, or Pepto-Bismol. Take as prescribed on the package. Eat foods high in soluble fiber, which slows diarrhea by absorbing liquid. In addition to the BRAT diet, these foods include oatmeal, cream-of-wheat, grits, and soft bread (not whole grain).

• • •

Avoid foods high in insoluble fiber, like the skins of vegetables and fruits. These foods can make diarrhea worse. Avoid milk products and greasy, high-fiber, or very sweet foods. They tend to aggravate diarrhea.

Many people taking the protease inhibitor nelfinavir (Viracept) experience diarrhea or loose stool. Try psyllium-husk powder (Metamucil or Konsyl). This is a natural, concentrated vegetable powder, not a laxative, nor even a medication. Mix one teaspoon of the powder with eight to ten ounces of water or juice and swallow. For best results, you should start taking psyllium three to four days before starting Viracept.

FATIGUE

Fatigue is a little more than garden-variety tiredness. Fatigue is a more profound tiredness that keeps you from doing the normal things in life and it's common during the adjustment period. You may feel weary or exhausted in a physical, emotional, or mental way. Your body, especially your arms and legs, may feel heavy. You may find it hard to concentrate or think clearly.

Rest and sleep are important, but don't sleep too much, this can decrease your energy level. In other words, the more you rest, the more tired you will feel. If you have trouble sleeping, talk to your doctor or nurse. Consider taking a "power nap" during the day for one hour or less.

Stay as active as you can. Try light exercise such as walking. You may find that you're most able to exercise early in the day. Try spreading your activities throughout the day. Let others help you with meals, housework, or errands.

If fatigue persists longer than four to six weeks, ask your doctor about anemia. Anemia means the blood has a low red blood cell count, and red blood cells are the vehicles that deliver oxygen to different parts of your body. When your body is short on oxygen, you feel fatigued. The HIV drug zidovudin or AZT (Retrovir) is notorious for causing anemia, especially in women.

Doctors are usually quick to dismiss fatigue as "something in your head," stress, or depression. If it persists, you'll need to become more assertive with your healthcare provider. If you are writing down symptoms in your health journal, you will be better able to describe in detail how fatigue is interfering with normal activities and ask specifically about your red blood cell count. There are treatments for both fatigue and anemia.

Allergic drug reactions

ABACAVIR (ZIAGEN)

About 3 to 5 percent of people who take the drug abacavir (Ziagen) have a potentially serious allergic reaction to it. This usually develops within two weeks of starting the drug. However, it can appear up to six weeks or more after starting. Signs of this reaction include fever, rash, cough, shortness of breath, or sore throat. If you develop any of these symptoms while taking abacavir, call your doctor immediately.

If you have an allergic reaction to abacavir, do not ever start taking it again. A few allergic patients who re-started abacavir had life-threatening reactions. If you ever stopped abacavir for any reason (for example, because you ran out), talk to your doctor before you start again. In rare cases, people who thought they weren't allergic had serious reactions when re-starting abacavir.

NEVIRAPINE (VIRAMUNE)

The most common side effect with nevirapine is skin rash, which occurs among 17 percent of patients who take the drug. The majority of severe rashes occurred within the first month of taking nevirapine. Most rashes are mild-to-moderate, but can be severe or life-threatening. If you develop any rash-like symptoms while taking nevirapine, contact your physician immediately, or go to an emergency room.

Every so often, side effects can become serious enough—or annoying enough—to require a switch one or more of the drugs in your combination. Switching a drug solely because of side effects may also save that drug as an option future. In fact, side effects from a drug at one time may not occur again if you take the drug later.

Believe me. I know how miserable it is when you're on the edge of vomiting all day long. It's not fun and it changes your entire outlook on life. Some days, it can feel as if life isn't worth living. But it is worth living and you'll put yourself in a really bad spot down the road by simply stopping one drug in your combination, or reducing the dose without talking first with your doctor and pharmacist.

On the bright side, there's good news for the not-too-distant future. Researchers are perfecting new tests that can measure the amount of drug your in blood. This means that your doctor will be able to better tailor drug dosing to an individual's needs and minimize side effects. These tests may also help provide better and long-lasting anti-HIV responses.

IN A SENTENCE:

> *You should expect some side effects from HIV treatment, but they'll likely subside with time.*

MONTH **11**

living

Planning
for Plan B

THE TELEPHONE rings. It's your doctor. He's calling to
say that your viral load is up. Suddenly it feels like the rug is
pulled from under you. Again.

A rising viral load while on HIV treatment usually means one
of three things: (1) your drug combination isn't working anymore, (2) you're not adhering to the drug combination, or
(3) you're experiencing a "viral blip," a transient and temporary
rise of viral load that's common and doesn't mean anything. The
problem is that all three scenarios start off in the same
fashion—your viral load begins to rise despite HIV treatment.

First off, don't panic. If you're on HIV treatment and you get
one viral load test that's higher than expected, it may not mean
a whole lot. However, if you get two or three viral load results
that consistently show an increase, that's a different story.

It's true that sometime during your treatment lifetime you
should expect to fail HIV drugs—or—the HIV drugs will fail
you. It happens both ways. Either way, there are still other
options. You may need to switch some drugs around. You may
need to adhere to your meds with more vigilance. You don't
want to let the situation spiral out of control, which ultimately
leads to more loss of immune function.

You'll have more options and more peace of mind by knowing your treatment options down the road. Imagine driving on an unfamiliar highway with only a half tank of gas. One option is to keep driving blindly. Perhaps you'll run across a gas station when you need one. Another option is to look at a map to get a sense of what's ahead. With a map, you can better plan your route. You might even enjoy the ride.

A rising viral load could just be a blip

Say you're tooting along on HIV treatment and everything is going well. Your T-cells are up and your viral load is less than 40 copies. Then, one day your doctor ruins your groove with the news that your viral load is up a bit. There's a chance this is just a viral blip, an intermittent spike of low-level virus that just happens in people on successful HIV treatment.

If your viral load had been undetectable (below 40 copies) and then blips, is not a bad sign, according to research. Viral blips are not associated with treatment failure and do not predict failure, at least in treatment-naïve people.

A viral blip is a viral load of more than 50 copies in someone who was previously was below 50 copies for an extended length of time. It's only a blip if the next viral load test shows the viral levels to be below 50 once again. Two consecutive viral load results above 200 copies is considered to be treatment failure, at least by most doctors. According to Daniel S. Berger, M.D., medical director of Northstar Medical Center in Chicago "even *two* viral loads above 50 may just be one blip that takes longer to come down."

There was a time when doctors and researchers blamed viral blips entirely on the patient not being adherent. Now, doctors know that blips can happen even if the patient is completely adherent to their meds. Doctors now think that blips may be caused by fluctuating levels of HIV drugs in the blood or that the virus is getting cleaned out from hard-to-reach areas of your body.

A rising viral load over time is not a blip

Don't sweat it over a one-time blip in viral load. However, if the blip doesn't go away, it becomes a different ballgame. "If sequential viral load testing shows a trend of increasing viral levels, and they are increasing to concerning levels—say they are 200, then 800, then 1,200, and then

1,500—obviously that's failing. Changing the regimen should be considered," says Berger.

"But if [one viral load test is] 200 or 300, I wouldn't necessarily say you're failing the regimen, especially if you're feeling well and not having any difficulty in taking the medication." Berger explained that when a viral load begins to climb in a patient, he inquires about the patient's adherence to meds.

"You want to be absolutely sure that you're taking the medications 100 percent of the time, not 80 or 85 percent of the time. That might be the difference," says Berger. "So you may not be failing the regimen, you may be just failing *taking* the regimen. In which case, if you get back on the wagon and take the medications 100 percent of the time, the viral levels usually come back down."

For better or worse, many people who test positive for HIV these days may not be as motivated as people were in the past. "There's this entire generation of people whose direct involvement with HIV was after the mid-1990s," says Bob Munk, an HIV advocate and operator of the AIDS InfoNet. "They never saw their friends get sick and die. So, they have a skewed risk-benefit assessment internally for anti-viral therapy. They don't really see the benefits with the same clarity that they see the side effects."

Berger concurs, adding that many people today are younger, in their late teens and early twenties. "They didn't see people during the 1980s and early 1990s walking around the street with their bones showing, looking like skeletons, and often with purple spots on their face, depicting hallmarks of Kaposi's sarcoma, and appearing very sickly," says Berger. "So they don't have a frame of reference or understand what it means to have AIDS."

Not being adherent isn't always your fault

"So I go get this new job and it's really demanding," says Alan G. "I'm not about to take my meds during a staff meeting. Try timing medicine and food at a Thanksgiving dinner. Imagine landing in Peru for work, while your luggage (and meds) land in Colombia. I'm a fairly organized guy, but I'm no Superman."

On one hand, we all know that treatment adherence is important. On the other hand, we are just human and sometimes we get tired, lazy, or forgetful. "A while back, my doctor asked if I missed doses of medicine. I said 'yes.' He looked disappointed, wrote something in my chart, and then delivered a four-minute speech that left me with anxiety and guilt," says Alan G.

"Now when my doc asks the same question, I think for a moment. 'Do I want the speech or not? I'm sure I miss a dose now and then, but I don't admit to it," he says. "It's just easier."

An acquaintance of mine pleads the fifth with his doctor as well. Not only does he miss meds for the usual reasons, but he occasionally takes extended drug and alcohol getaways. He's a party boy and likes circuit parties where it's easy to buy underground drugs such as cocaine, Special K, Ecstasy, or Crystal (a.k.a. methamphetamine). He knows it's unwise to mix HIV meds with street drugs, so he opts for the street drugs and lies to his doctor.

But lying to your doctor is also lying to yourself. If you've made the decision to start HIV treatment, but you find yourself telling white lies to your doctor, the problem just might be with your doctor. "Find a physician who you can be very comfortable with, that you can tell everything to, not one that you have to hide things from," advises Berger.

Research shows that patients treated by doctors with more HIV experience tend to fare a little better. Research also shows that it's unlikely you'll be 100 percent adherent to your meds over the course of years. So it's up to your doctor to match the right drug combination to the right patient.

"See a physician that has experience with HIV, that has been doing this for a long time, not somebody that has a few patients that happen to be HIV-positive," says Berger. "I try to make it very easy, because if I make it easy for the patient, then he or she is more apt to continue taking or adhere to the medication regimen. By doing so, it will remain effective for a lot longer than not."

"Patients often ask me, how long will this last? They've heard that perhaps eighteen months is the average time that these regimens last," says Berger. "Some studies have been done to see what the average time was on the initial regimen. I wonder about which regimens these patients were initially offered. Were they put on difficult regimens?"

Berger explains that he steers away from offering three-times-a-day regimens or regimens that require an empty stomach four times a day. "I don't know how physicians can actually put a person on such a regimen," says Berger. "What kind of thought process was involved when a physician puts a patient on a regimen that's difficult to take and potentially has more side effects?"

"Ideally, people should be able to trust their doc," says Munk. "But plenty of people have raised questions about physicians who are intimately involved in researching new products and whether they are sufficiently objective or get swept in the enthusiasm. That's certainly what I'd like to think, that just they're get swept up in the enthusiasm."

The bottom line is that a blip or short-term rise in viral load is probably not reason for concern. "If patients do remain on the regimen, they can go far beyond what has been shown in some statistically in studies," says Berger. "I have patients who have been on their original regimens for years."

IN A SENTENCE:

A temporary rise in viral load while on HIV treatment can mean many things.

learning

If Treatment Fails

IF YOUR HIV viral load was below 40 or 50 copies for an extended period, and then it jumps higher on two consecutive occasions, most doctors would agree this to be treatment failure, assuming viral blips or adherence can be ruled out.

If you are experiencing treatment failure, at the end of the day, the problem is resistance. HIV has become resistant to one or all of the drugs in your combination. Think of the virus as a forest fire and your three-drug combo as three different fire roads. For whatever reason, the fire jumped at least one of the roads and is now burning away on the other side.

Keep in mind that once you've taken HIV meds, you lose the title "treatment naïve." It goes to someone else. Your new category: "treatment experienced." If you've ever taken HIV drugs, you're considered treatment experienced. Goals for those with extensive treatment experience can differ somewhat from those who are drug naïve.

One man's failure is another man's success

HIV treatment changes fast, according to Daniel S. Berger, M.D., medical director of Northstar Medical. "It continues to shift with every passing year. HIV treatment is continuing to evolve, not from decade to decade—but month to month and week to week."

For example, today's definition of "treatment failure" is very different from what it was ten years ago. At one time, "treatment failure" meant an AIDS-defining opportunistic infection. Today, it means two consecutive viral loads above 50 copies or T-cells below a specific threshold, say 200.

To put it another way, *treatment failure* is really just an artificial milestone, agreed upon by you and your doctor. Some people can negotiate with their doctors to agree on what constitutes treatment failure, says Bob Munk. "Say you're a person who would get freaked out about sunken cheeks, then have an agreement with your doc, that 'we'll try this regimen until I start seeing signs of sunken cheeks, then we're going to switch to something else.'"

Expectations for second-line treatment should be lower

Your expectation should be a little less for a second-line treatment compared to a first-line regimen. If you're treatment experienced or have resistance, you might not be able to get your viral load to undetectable; it may not be practical. In which case, the goals become to preserve your immune functioning and to avoid any complications from HIV, mainly opportunistic infections and other metabolic problems.

"For a person who is highly exposed [to treatment] or already has a lot of resistant mutations, you expect for their viral load not to remain fully suppressed," says Berger. "You can't put patients on [too many drugs] just to try to drive the viral load down because that's toxic. So for patients who are highly experienced, our goals of treatment are to preserve their [T-cells] and their immune system, to preserve their quality of life. Additionally we try to reduce the propensity of side effects, reduce the potential for the development of metabolic problems and lipodystrophy while reducing the risks for other long-term complications."

So the goals for the drug-naïve patient and treatment-experienced patient are somewhat different, with the focus for treatment-experienced on quality of life and reducing side effects, while maintaining or enhancing immune function."

Treatment interruptions between regimens are dicey

If your first-line HIV treatment has failed, you might consider taking a temporary break from all anti-HIV drugs. Treatment interruptions are being studied in a range of settings, however, mostly for people with extensive treatment experience. During a treatment interruption, sometimes the virus reverts to the old, non-resistant type. Some doctors say this can lead to a better response for new regimens. "Thus for the highly experienced patient with few alternatives, this option definitely needs to be placed on the table," says Berger.

A recent case report suggested that long treatment interruption may clear resistant HIV, while another study suggests that resistant HIV persists even in the absence of treatment. What's clear, at this point, is that treatment interruptions can cause significant decreases of T-cells and increases in viral load.

"I think that's something that hasn't been completely worked out yet," says Berger. "We don't know how often or how long a treatment interruption should occur. We don't know all the strategies that are possible. We do know that a lot of factors can contribute to [treatment] failure.

"Not only is [the problem] resistant mutations, but sometimes it's poor or lower drug absorption, maybe the presence of compartments where drugs can't get into to achieve the appropriate levels needed to suppress the virus," says Berger. "If those are the problems, then going off treatment won't solve that part of the problem."

Resistance testing helps you make better choices about drugs

You don't really need to know exactly *how* resistance tests work, in order to understand what it means. There are two types of tests: **genotypic** and **phenotypic.**

Genotypic tests use a sample of your blood to identify mutations in the virus that are resistant to specific drugs. Genotypic tests use DNA, special chemicals, and computers to produce a snapshot of the virus that's inside you and only you. The snapshot is a picture of the "resistance mutations" that your virus has created to survive.

These mutations are given names, such as "M41" or "184V." For example, if you have an M41 mutation it might mean that Drug A will no longer work for you. On the other hand, if you have a 184V mutation, it might mean that both Drug A and Drug B won't work. Interpreting mutations is complicated and getting more so every day.

Phenotype tests use a sample of your blood. But this time, HIV is grown in your laboratory sample and it's then tested against different HIV drugs to what works and what doesn't.

"I think genotypic testing is too limited," notes Berger. "A genotypic test gives you the mutations that can be isolated from a particular patient, but

Case Study:
What Bob Would Do

HIV DRUGS change over time. Individuals are different. Matching the right drugs to the right person is a two-way street between physician and a patient. As a patient, you don't need to know everything about every drug. That's your doctor's job. For your part, it helps to have a sense the big picture.

People make different decisions when it comes to HIV treatment. To give you a feel for your options, consider the case of Bob. Bob is a regular guy, easily confused by the dozens of drugs from which to construct a HIV treatment regimen.

BOB'S FIRST STEP

When Bob was deciding whether or not to start HIV treatment, his priority was convenience. He didn't want treatment to interfere with his daily activities. Working with his doctor, he looked at all his possibilities:

Protease inhibitors (PIs)	Non-nucleoside reverse transcriptase inhibitors (non-nukes)	Nucleoside reverse transcriptase inhibitors (nukes)
Fortovase (saquinavir)	Viramune (nevirapine)	Retrovir (zidovudine)
Norvir (ritonavir)	Sustiva (efavirenz)	Epivir (lamivudine)
Crixivan (indinavir)	Rescriptor (delavirdine)	Videx EC (didanosine)
Viracept (nelfinavir)		Zerit (stavudine)
Agenerase (amprenavir)		Ziagen (abacavir)
Kaletra (lopinavir/ritonavir)		Viread (tenofovir)
Reyataz (atazanavir)		Coviracil (emtricitabine)
tipranavir		

BOB'S CHOOSES . . .

Bob and his doctor decided to go with Trizivir, which is a combination of abacavir, zidovudine, and lamivudine formulated into one pill, taken twice a day. They also knew that this strategy spared two drug classes for the future: protease inhibitors and non-nukes.

	Drug 1	Drug 2	Drug 3
PI			
Nuke	abacavir	zidovudine	lamivudine
Non-nuke			

Eight months later, after Bob saw an initial drop in viral load, his virus levels began to increase over time. Bob suspects this happened because he sometimes forgot his pills on the weekends.

CONSTRUCTING A SECOND-LINE TREATMENT FOR BOB

Over time, Bob's T-cells begin to decrease and he figures it's time to start HIV treatment once again. Since Bob still has two new drug classes to choose from, he and his doctor decide to go with a "non-nuke based" regimen with efavirenz, tenofovir, and emtricitabine. Bob's drug archive now includes the drugs he's already used.

	Drug 1	Drug 2	Drug 3
PI			
Nuke		tenofovir	emtricitabine
Non-nuke	efavirenz		

Bob's drug archive would be: abacavir, zidovudine, and lamivudine.

THIRD-LINE TREATMENT FOR BOB

Although Bob's second-line treatment seems to be holding up, he prefers to keep his options open for the future. Both Bob and his doctor agree that if Bob were to fail second-line treatment, one viable option would be the following:

	Drug 1	Drug 2	Drug 3
PI	atazanavir		
Nuke		didanosine	stavudine
Non-nuke			

Bob's drug archive would be: abacavir, zidovudine, lamivudine, efavirenz, tenofovir, and emtricitabine.

if the physician doesn't completely understand how to interpret the results, they can easily be misinterpreted. The physician may be falsely interpreting [the results], when, in fact, the patient does have a lot of options."

A recent study of healthcare professionals caring for people with HIV found that only about a quarter of them can accurately match the majority of genotypic HIV resistance mutations to the drug class affected. Guidelines exist to recommend the use of genotypic testing for HIV patients, but proper interpretation of the results is harder to come by.

The International AIDS Society-USA provides doctors with a resistance mutation chart for interpreting genotyping results (online at http://www.iasusa.org). The chart is continuously updated and provides user notes to explain the significance of specific mutations.

"Virlogic does have a test called a PhenoSense GT, which combines the two tests," says Berger. "They also provide for free a lab test called a viral 'replicative capacity.' When HIV becomes resistant to some drugs, it also loses some of its strength or 'fitness.' In other words, although viral loads persist in the blood, a reduced replicative capacity indicates that the virus is crippled and has a reduced ability to kill T-cells." Research has shown that measuring viral fitness can provide valuable information that can guide you and your healthcare provider in making better treatment decisions. "In other words, even if there's resistance—if the [viral fitness] is low—you're more likely to maintain immune function."

Second-line treatment is a second chance to control the virus

"It's like a chess game. You always have to think a couple of moves in advance," says Berger. "Treatments are limited, but there's going be a move, a move after that, and a move after that. Our treatment approach has evolved in this way out of necessity, ensuring that patients have as many later options as possible."

Berger explains that certain medications have the potential for causing other medications to be ruled out in the future. In other words, Drug A can rule out Drug B at a later time. This sequence, he says, has to be carefully considered.

Optimism among the HIV community has come with the introduction of newer classes of drugs, such as the fusion inhibitors, including Fuzeon (enfuvirtide). However, the optimism is primary for **salvage therapy**, which is a last-ditch—but potent—attempt to snuff out the virus.

"I'm very forthright and honest with patients that if they wanted to explore [Fuzeon], it's open," says Berger. "But they need to understand that the drug needs to be self-injected twice daily and it's very expensive. For people who are at a later stage and have exhausted options, it's a very important drug and should not be overlooked. It can be a lifesaving drug, but it has its limitations. Longer-acting fusion inhibitors, which require less frequent injections, are being developed, and an oral entry inhibitor being developed by Schering Plough is also currently in the pipeline. The landscape of HIV treatment is a dynamic entity with continuous evolution and change. Therefore, patients can be more hopeful about the future."

IN A SENTENCE:

> *If treatment failure occurs, physician experience and resistance testing can be critical to preserve immune function and reduce side effects.*

MONTH **12**

living

Having Children

YOU'RE HUMAN first. After that, you're either a man or a woman. Then comes being straight, gay, or falling somewhere in between. But at the end of the day, you'll always be human first.

Because you're human, you were built to survive. This survival instinct is weaved into your DNA, cells, emotions, and your everyday behavior. But when there's no immediate threat to your well-being, you, like all humans, start looking around for something more.

Eventually, you'll understand that HIV is no longer a threat to you. Your planning, healthy behaviors, medical care, treatment strategies, adherence to medication will all come together and tip the scales toward feeling safe and reasonably assured about your future. You'll start to feel like a regular human being again.

There was a time when having HIV meant *not* having children. Doctors and health officials generally agreed that people with HIV wouldn't live long enough to care for children. That was when—for HIV-positive women—the high risk of passing the virus to the baby during delivery was unacceptable. For HIV-positive men, the central issue was the unacceptable risk of passing the virus to the mother.

• • •

Those obstacles have been overcome. Those days are gone. And don't let anybody tell you otherwise. The right to procreate is central to personal identity, dignity, and to the meaning of one's life.

Now, whether you actually want children is a different matter. That decision is up to you. Just know that if you decide that you do want children, it *is* possible.

Here's a look at why this consensus has changed over the years, a few considerations to keep in mind, and some specific suggestions on how to make it all happen—for both women and for men.

Women with HIV can safely have healthy children

"If a woman wants to have children, she can. HIV is not going to stop her from having children," says Precious J., of Women Alive, an AIDS service organization in Los Angeles, California. "Thank God, we do have medication that can reduce the transmission of HIV to the baby."

Years ago, before effective treatment for HIV, the risk of a woman passing the virus to her child during pregnancy was as high as 30 percent. Today, through the judicious use of HIV treatment, delivery by cesarean section, and avoidance of breast-feeding, this risk is now less than 2 percent—a risk to the baby that's comparable to HIV-negative women over the age of 40, or those with diabetes.

Recent studies also show that HIV-positive women who get pregnant do not get any sicker than those who are not pregnant. That is, becoming pregnant does not appear to be dangerous to the health of an HIV-positive woman.

Potential harmful effects to the baby by HIV treatment—taken by the mother during pregnancy—remain a concern. For many years, it was common for pregnant women to take zidovudine (Retrovir) alone. However, a recent study of women with HIV who gave birth showed a dramatic change in the individual medications taken by women during pregnancy.

The study showed that the use of zidovudine decreased from 96 percent during the early 1990s to only 6 percent during 2001. During the same time, use of three-drug regimens that included a protease inhibitor increased to 41 percent, and regimens that included a non-nucleoside reverse transcriptase inhibitors (non-nuke) increased to 43 percent.

Researchers have studied the use of HIV treatment during the first, second, and third trimesters of pregnancy and observed no increase in birth defects. They concluded that, while the results are preliminary, this research does provide "some reassurance" regarding the trends of using three-drug combinations during pregnancy.

However, they also cautioned that there's not enough long-term research about the risks of some specific drugs. Either way, the research is helpful in discussing options for women undergoing HIV treatment who are considering pregnancy. It should be noted that efavirenz (Sustiva) has been shown to cause birth defects in animals.

Some doctors are rethinking the generally supported view that the use of a cesarean ("C") section to reduce the possibility of transmitting the virus from mother to child during labor. In a presentation at a recent AIDS conference, Karen P. Beckerman, M.D., director of the Bay Area Perinatal AIDS Center at the University of California, San Francisco, suggested that there's not enough evidence to support the notion that healthy HIV-infected pregnant women should routinely be offered C-sections. Clearly, more research is needed.

Can women with HIV create a family? "Yes, and I've seen it," says Jelka Jonker, a counselor and therapist at AIDS Project Los Angeles. However, she said that women should first go through all the stages of emotions that come with a new diagnosis of HIV. They need to become comfortable themselves first.

There are going to be obstacles. According to Jonker, HIV-positive women have a harder time finding a partner. "Say a woman finds somebody and they decide to have children, a lot of people are going to be very judgmental. Some people think 'how can you be so selfish?' Or, 'you might not live that long.' So it's not easy. You have to be a really strong person to overcome all of that."

Men want children—whether they verbalize it or not

Straight or gay, almost every man values the idea of having offspring, his own flesh and blood, whether he verbalizes it or not. Men are human first and all humans are imbedded with the desire to procreate. Men who seek the same gender for sexual expression are still following the same natural human instincts for procreation as those who prefer the opposite gender.

"The very first thought I had when I tested positive was that I'd never have kids," says Mark H. "I don't know why, but that part bothered me the most."

With new technology, HIV-positive men can father children without passing on the virus. Fertility researchers have developed a technique called "sperm washing" where sperm is isolated from fluid and white blood cells—the most likely place where HIV hides. If doctors don't find HIV in the sperm sample, then it is joined with an egg through *in vitro* fertilization.

In vitro fertilization is a process that involves retrieving eggs from ovaries, placing them in special solutions, and combining the sperm and eggs in a dish. The resulting embryos are placed in an incubator where they're nourished until maturity. At the appropriate time, the pre-embryos are removed from the dish and replaced in the uterus, where they continue on with normal fetal development.

Only a handful of fertility centers in the United States have experience with these techniques, which have given life to many healthy, HIV-negative children as well as protected their mothers from the virus. Ideal candidates are men with low or undetectable levels of HIV.

Help with fertility is there if you want it

The American Society for Reproductive Medicine (ASRM) now offers new guidelines for treating infertility in people with HIV. The guidelines examine several different scenarios and issues. The document offers information for different situations, such as when one partner only has HIV or when both partners have HIV.

According to the ASRM, doctors who practice reproductive medicine should deny treatment to individuals with HIV. Ethically and legally, fertility doctors have the same obligation to treat patients with HIV as they do patients with any other chronic illness. When a clinic lacks the skills and facilities to manage people with HIV, the clinic should provide a referral to another clinic that has these resources.

"With the development of new techniques and treatment protocols, we're able now to help HIV-positive patients have children while minimizing the risks they face," says William Keye, Jr., M.D., president of the American Society of Reproductive Medicine.

"A lot of times in our society, we always say what people should do— until we are in that position—and then we should do something different," says Rosetta M., who also works in the health education field. However, she adds, generally people in the United States don't take advantage of adoption or becoming a foster parent. Still, she contends that people with HIV should have the right to procreate.

"HIV is like any other disease or genetic condition, you don't know what the future holds," says Rosetta M. If people with HIV "should not" have kids, she argues, then if you're forced to work two jobs and can't stay home, you shouldn't have kids either. If you have herpes, you shouldn't have kids.

FOR MORE INFORMATION ON PREGNANCY AND HIV

American Society for Reproductive Medicine
1209 Montgomery Highway
Birmingham, Alabama 35216
(205) 978-5000

Jones Institute for Reproductive Medicine
601 Colley Ave
Norfolk, VA 23507
(800) 515-6637

IN A SENTENCE:

It is possible to safely have healthy children

learning

Keep Moving Forward

SO WHAT does the future look like for HIV? It's hard to say. Finding a cure for HIV may be possible in our lifetime. After all, there were few effective treatments before 1996, and now there are many effective treatments available. In looking forward, it's hard to predict what might happen. Conventional wisdom may suddenly shift. More research will become available with time. New drugs, better combinations, novel blood tests, and vaccines will be invented. HIV treatment is an evolving science.

New and better drugs coming down the pipeline is good reason for optimism, according to Anthony Fauci, M.D., director of the National Institute of Allergy and Infectious Diseases. He notes that over the next few years, new HIV drugs will be developed that specifically target HIV in different ways than the older drugs.

The future of HIV medicine, Fauci says, will "skirt away from the protease reverse transcriptase inhibitors and common [cross resistant] prototype drugs." It's a work in progress—that's the good news and the bad news. It's not absolute now."

So how do you keep track of HIV medicine as it changes over time? First, decide if it's even worth your time. Everyone is different. Some people choose only to learn about HIV treatment as they need it, so they can get on with the business of living. Other people monitor newsletters and Web sites on occasion. A few get more involved by "giving back" or volunteering.

Giving back can mean many things

"I don't think there's an obligation to give back," says Rosetta M., who also works in the health education field. "First, figure out where you are emotionally, before you try to branch out and give pieces of yourself away. I think there are other ways people can give back, by living healthy—living a prosperous life—and I don't mean financial.

"Being happy, that's giving back," says Rosetta. "Then there's one less miserable bitch walking around. Just being able to walk outside and say hi to somebody else—'good morning' and smile or whatever—you're giving back."

With time, some people with HIV get involved in things that are meaningful for them. "If you know that you've been helped and you've gone through all those emotions—and if you came out as a better person—it can change people's attitude toward life," says Jelke Jonker, a counselor at AIDS Project Los Angeles.

"People have told me that being HIV-positive has changed their life in a better way because they now have a more productive attitude toward life. Obviously, that's not true for everybody. But a lot of people have told me that."

Some people are driven by civic or moral duty so they turn outward and gain satisfaction from helping others. Other people are driven more out of self-interest and ask, "What's in it for me?" Humans are complicated beings; we're both selfless and selfish at the same time.

If you've had some good fortune along the way, if somebody took you under their wing at some point, then I think you owe a little something. Think of it as "fee for services" if that suits you better.

So how do you pay it forward? One way is to volunteer at an AIDS service organization, or become a facilitator for people who are newly diagnosed, or just be nice to other people. "What better way to give back for the things you have received when you needed them?" says Jonker.

Keeping up with the details of HIV can't hurt

Most people with HIV get their treatment news from their doctor, newsletters, or the Internet. In all three cases, you might not be able to judge the quality of the information you are getting from these sources. One way is to diversify your sources of information. For example, you might learn something in a newsletter and then ask your doctor for his thoughts on the same subject. Here's a look at some reliable and trustworthy sources of information:

If activism inspires you

WANT TO do something but you don't know how to start? Here's a short list of key organizations involved with HIV politics and policy.

AIDS ACTION

AIDS Action is a political group that keeps tabs on national policies regarding HIV. In a sense, the group educates and "motivates" elected officials so that people with HIV are represented on a national level.

AIDS Action
1906 Sunderland Place NW
Washington, DC 20036
(202) 530-8030

SURVIVE AIDS

Survive AIDS is the new name for what was once called ACT UP Golden Gate. It is a grassroots, all-volunteer group of individuals in San Francisco, California, who work in different ways to ensure adequate funding and resources for the care, treatment, and prevention of HIV.

Survive AIDS
584 Castro Street, PMB 542
San Francisco, CA 94114
(415) 252-9200
http://www.surviveaids.org

ACT UP NEW YORK

ACT UP is a diverse, non-partisan group of individuals committed to direct action to end the AIDS crisis. The group's motto: "Our job is not to be invited to coffee or to schmooze at a cocktail party. Our job is to make change happen as fast as possible and direct action works for that."

ACT UP/New York
332 Bleecker St. Suite G5
New York, NY 10014
(212) 966-4873
http://www.actupny.org

POZ MAGAZINE

Poz is a four-color glossy magazine published in New York City. *Poz* is engaging, accessible, and isn't homework. It's very conversational, pleasing to look at, and tuned into culture and lifestyle issues. The magazine is free to people who are HIV-positive and who cannot afford a subscription—one year of 12 issues is $19.97. (It's well worth the money.) Make sure you specifically request that the company doesn't make your name available to other groups.

Poz magazine
One Little West 12th Street
New York, NY 10014
(800) 973-2376
Outside U.S., (815) 734-1292
http://www.poz.com

POSITIVELY AWARE

Positively Aware is magazine-like in that it's printed in four-color, but it feels and reads more like a "grassroots," treatment-focused publication. Given the technical nature of HIV treatment, *Positively Aware* offers a respectable choice of plain-language articles and commentary. The publication produces an annual "drug guide" that is particularly noteworthy.

Positively Aware
Test Positive Aware Network
5537 N. Broadway Street
Chicago, IL 60640-1405
(773) 989-9400
http://www.tpan.com

AIDS INFONET.ORG

AIDS InfoNet is a Web site originally designed to make information on HIV services and treatments easily accessible in English and Spanish for residents of New Mexico. However, the Web site has become widely acclaimed for its non-technical fact sheets, which are updated frequently to reflect advances in medicine, and are available in both English and Spanish.

New Mexico AIDS InfoNet
PO Box 810
Arroyo Seco, NM 87514
http://www.aidsinfonet.org

HIVandHepatitis.com

HIVandHepatitis.com is a Web site based in San Francisco, California. It offers a steady stream of accurate, timely, and cutting-edge information about treatment for HIV, hep B, and hep C. It's especially unique in that issues related to co-infections are well covered.

> *HIVandHepatitis.com*
> PO Box 14288
> San Francisco, CA 94114
> http://www.HIVandHepatitis.com

NATAP.org

NATAP is a New York-based non-profit organization that operates a no-nonsense Web site focused primarily on HIV and hep C treatment. The Web site offers the latest developments in treatment with a clear commitment to objectivity and deciphering fact from the claims of the pharmaceutical companies.

> *NATAP*
> 580 Broadway, Suite 1010
> New York, NY 10012
> (212) 219-0106
> http://www.natap.org

You are now armed for life

Now you are armed with the knowledge and the tools you need to survive HIV. You have an understanding of the virus, your own emotions, getting proper medical care, sexually transmitted diseases, mental health, nutrition, exercise, treatment strategies, and a dose of hope for the future. The choice to act on this knowledge is now your own. Like it or not, you're in control. You can make smart choices over time. Or not. Better choices over time spin the odds in your favor. The choice is yours.

IN A SENTENCE:

> *Giving back and staying connected to HIV organizations, newsletters, and Web sites can help you make better choices in the future.*

Glossary

ACUTE INFECTION: The phase of HIV infection when the blood contains many viral particles that spread throughout the body, seeding themselves in various organs, particularly the lymphoid tissues.

"AIDS" COCKTAIL: Another name for **combination therapy.**

AMPHETAMINE: Drugs that speed up the way your body works. They make your heart work faster, and they pump adrenaline into the system. The user feels more energetic, cheerful, and confident, and because of these effects there is a high risk of psychological dependence.

ANGIOTENSIN CONVERTING ENZYME (ACE) INHIBITORS: Medications that lower blood pressure and are commonly prescribed for the treatment of high blood pressure (hypertension).

ANILINGUS: Erotic stimulation achieved by contact between mouth and anus.

ANTIRETROVIRALS: Drugs that work by interfering with the HIV life cycle. When used in combination, these medications reduce the amount of virus in the blood and help to delay the progress of disease.

ANTIVIRALS: Drugs that work by changing the genetic material of the host cell so that the virus cannot use the host's genetic material as efficiently.

ANXIETY: An emotional state in which people feel uneasy, apprehensive, or fearful.

ASPARTATE TRANSAMINASE (AST): A type of enzyme that is found in blood serum and certain body tissues, especially the heart and the liver.

ASPERGILLOSIS: An infection with, or disease caused by, molds.

ASYMPTOMATIC SHEDDING: Occurs when the herpes virus is released in genital secretions or on the skin when the sores or lesions that mark an active genital herpes outbreak are absent, and is a major vehicle of transmission of the genital herpes virus.

BAREBACKING: Generally refers to gay men engaging in unprotected anal intercourse.

BENZODIAZEPINE: A class of commonly prescribed tranquilizers that can cause addiction.

bDNA (BRANCHED DNA): A test that combines a material that gives off light with the sample. This material connects with the HIV particles. The amount of light is measured and converted to a viral count.

BUSPIRONE (BuSPAR): A medication that relieves anxiety with minimal sedation, minimal muscle relaxation, and no addiction potential.

CANDIDIASIS (THRUSH, YEAST INFECTION): A fungal infection characterized by white patches in the mouth, difficulty swallowing, and, in women, vaginal irritation and thick, white discharge.

CD4 CELL: One of the two main types of T-cells, also known as "helper" cells, which leads the attack against infections.

COMBINATION THERAPY: Using more than one drug at a time.

CUNNILINGUS: Oral stimulation of the vulva or clitoris.

DENTAL DAM: A small sheet of latex which acts as a barrier between the vagina or anus and the mouth.

DIABETES MELLITUS: A condition characterized by raised concentration of sugar in the blood and urine, due to problems with the production or action of insulin.

DIACETYLMORPHINE: A highly addictive morphine derivative.

DISASSOCIATION: The separation of whole segments of the personality (as in multiple personality) or of discrete mental processes (as in the schizophrenia) from the mainstream of consciousness or of behavior.

DNA: Deoxyribonucleic acid, the material in the nucleus of a cell where genetic information is stored.

DYSPLASIA: An abnormal growth or development of organs or cells.

ECSTASY: A synthetic amphetamine analogue used illicitly for its mood-enhancing and hallucinogenic properties.

EPISODIC THERAPY: Taking medication only during an outbreak to speed healing.

GENOTYPIC: A type of drug resistance testing that directly exposes a person's virus to antiviral drugs to determine how much of the drug is required to block viral activity.

GLUCOSE: A form of sugar found in the bloodstream. All sugars and starches are converted into glucose before they are absorbed.

HEPATITIS C VIRUS (HVC): A form of liver inflammation that causes rapidly developing and often chronic disease.

HIGHLY ACTIVE ANTIRETROVIRAL THERAPY (HAART): A term used to describe anti-HIV combination therapy with three or more drugs.

HUMAN PAPILLOMA VIRUS (HPV): A group of wart-causing viruses which are also responsible for cancer of the cervix and some anal cancers.

HYPOCHONDRIA: Extreme depression of the mind and spirit often centered on imaginary physical ailments.

KAPOSI'S SARCOMA: A cancer characterized by red or purple blotches on the skin or mucous membranes; may also affect internal organs.

LIPODYSTROPHY: A disruption to the way the body produces, uses, and distributes fat among people taking anti-HIV therapy.

LIPOHYPERTROPHY: Abnormal fat gains that usually occur around the gut, waist, and back of the neck.

LOG: Short for logarithm, a scale of measurement often used when describing viral load. A one-log change is a ten-fold change, such as from 100 to 10. A two-log change is a one hundred-fold change, such as from 1,000 to 10.

METHAMPHETAMINE: A drug that works directly on the brain and spinal cord by interfering with normal neurotransmission. Neurotransmitters are chemical substances naturally produced within nerve cells used to communicate with each other and send messages to influence and regulate our thinking and all other systems throughout the body.

METHYLENEDIOXYMETHAMPHETAMINE (MDMA): See Ecstasy.

MONOAMINE OXIDASE INHIBITORS (MAOIs): Medicines that relieve certain types of mental depression.

NONOXYNOL-9: A spermicide used in contraceptive products.

OPPORTUNISTIC INFECTIONS: Specific infections that cause disease in someone with a damaged immune system.

PARTIAL SEROTONIN REUPTAKE INHIBITORS: A group of chemically unique antidepressant drugs that are effective in depression, bulimia nervosa, obsessive compulsive disorder, anorexia nervosa, panic disorder, pain associated with diabetic neuropathy and for premenstrual syndrome.

PATHOGENESIS: The origination and development of a disease.

PHENOTYPIC: A type of drug resistance testing that measures the amount of drug needed to suppress the growth of HIV in a laboratory setting.

PILL BURDEN: The number of pills you're required to take each day as part of your HIV drug therapy.

PNEUMOCYSTIS CARINII PNEUMONIA (PCP): A parasite that infects the lungs, causing fever, dry cough, shortness of breath. PCP is an AIDS-defining illness.

PCR (POLYMERASE CHAIN REACTION): A test that uses an enzyme to multiply the HIV in the blood sample. Then a chemical reaction marks the virus. The markers are measured and used to calculate the amount of virus.

PRODROME: A symptom of disease that warns you of its presence.

PROTEASE INHIBITOR (PI): Family of antiretrovirals that target the protease enzyme. Includes amprenavir, indinavir, lopinavir, ritonavir, saquinavir, nelfinavir, and atazanavir.

PSYCHOTHERAPY: Treatment of mental or emotional disorder or of related bodily ills by psychological means.

QI: An Eastern medicine term for the body's flow of energy.

RETROVIRUS: Family of viruses to which HIV belongs, that are distinguished by their use of RNA.

RNA: Ribonucleic acid, the form in which HIV stores its genetic material.

SALVAGE THERAPY: A course of action for people who have become fully or partially resistant to current drugs and are seeking drugs in new classes, older drugs to recycle, and other treatment strategies that may slow HIV and make their bodies' immune systems run efficiently again.

SEDATIVE: An agent or a drug having a soothing, calming, or tranquilizing effect.

SEROTONIN: A neurotransmitter involved in many behaviors, including human mood disorders and aggressive behaviors.

SEXUALLY TRANSMITTED DISEASE (STD): Any of various diseases transmitted by direct sexual contact that include venereal diseases (as syphilis, gonorrhea, and chancroid) and other diseases (as hepatitis A, hepatitis B, giardiasis, and AIDS) that are often or sometimes contracted by other than sexual means.

SURROGATE MARKERS: An indirect indicater of something, such as measuring viral load to assess the treament effect of a drug.

SUPPRESSIVE THERAPY: Taking an antiviral medication daily as a preventative measure, to keep HSV in check, reduce flare-ups, and lessen symptoms.

T-CELLS: A type of lymphocyte (white blood cell) that constitutes an important part of the immune system.

TETRAHYDROCANNABINOL (THC): A physiologically active chemical from hemp plant resin that is the chief intoxicant in marijuana.

TRICYCLICS: Antidepressants that relieve mental depression.

VIRAL LOAD: The amount of HIV virus in the blood.

Bibliography

Day 1: Living

1. Hogg, R., et al. "Improved Survival Among HIV-infected Individuals Following Initiation of Antiretroviral Therapy." *Journal of the American Medical Association* 1998; 279: 450–454.
2. Palella, F., et al. "Declining Morbidity and Mortality Among Patients with Advanced Human Immunodeficiency Virus Infection." *New England Journal of Medicine* 1998; 338: 853–860.
3. Smith, R. (Editor). *Encyclopedia of AIDS: A Social, Political, Cultural, and Scientific Record of the HIV Epidemic.* New York: Penguin, 2001.

Day 2: Learning

1. Samet, J., et al. "Trillion Virion Delay: Time From Testing Positive for HIV to Presentation for Primary Care." *Archives of Internal Medicine* 1998; 158: 734–740.
2. Leserman, J., et al. "Impact of stressful life events, depression, social support, coping, and cortisol on progression to AIDS." *American Journal of Psychiatry* 2000 Aug; 157(8):1221–8.
3. Canadian Psychiatric Association, *HIV & Psychiatry: A Training and Resource Manual.* Ottawa, Ontario: 2000.
4. Power, R., et al. "Self-disclosure of HIV serostatus in relation to depression and social support." Abstract. XIV International AIDS Conference, Barcelona, Spain, 2002.

Day 3: Living

1. Smith, R. (Editor). *Encyclopedia of AIDS: A Social, Political, Cultural, and Scientific Record of the HIV Epidemic.* New York: Penguin, 2001.
2. Centers for Disease Control & Prevention. "Preventing Infections from Pets: A Guide for People with HIV Infection." Fact Sheet. June 1999.
3. Gao, F., et al. "Origin of HIV-1 in the chimpanzee Pan troglodytes troglodytes." *Nature* 1999; 397: 436–41.
4. Weis, R., Wrangham, RW., "From Pan to pandemic." *Nature* 397, 385–6 (1999).
5. Zhu, T., et al. "An African HIV-1 Sequence from 1959 and Implications for the Origin of the Epidemic." *Nature* (02/05/98) Vol. 391, No. 6667, P. 594.
6. Centers for Disease Control & Prevention. "Questions and Answers: HIV is the Cause of AIDS." Fact Sheet. February, 2001.
7. Centers for Disease Control & Prevention. "How is HIV passed from one person to another?" Fact Sheet. November, 1998.
8. Safren, S., et al. "Predictors of Psychological Well-Being in a Diverse Sample of HIV-Positive Patients Receiving Highly Active Antiretroviral Therapy." *Psychosomatics* 2002; 43: 478–485.
9. Raymond, S. (Editor). *Encyclopedia of AIDS: A Social, Political, Cultural, and Scientific Record of the HIV Epidemic.* New York: Penguin, 2001.

Day 3: Learning

1. Agency for Healthcare Research and Quality by the Research Triangle Institute-University of North Carolina at Chapel Hill Evidence-based Practice Center. "Management of Dental Patients Who Are HIV Positive." Evidence Report/Technology Assessment No. 37.

Day 4: Living

1. Herek, G., Capitanio, J., Widaman, K. "HIV-related stigma and knowledge in the United States: prevalence and trends, 1991–1999." *American Journal of Public Health* 2002 Mar; 92(3):371–7.

Day 4: Learning

1. Harold, K. "An 83-Year-Old Woman with Chronic Illness and Strong Religious Beliefs." *Journal of the American Medical Association* 2002; 288:487–493.
2. Ironson, G., et al. "The Ironson-woods Spirituality/Religiousness Index is associated with long survival, health behaviors, less distress, and low cortisol in people with HIV/AIDS. *Ann Behav Med* 2002 Winter; 24(1):34–48.
3. Melbourne, K. "The Impact of Religion on Adherence with Antiretrovirals." *Journal of the Association of Nurses in AIDS Care* (05/99–06/99) Vol. 10, No. 3, P. 99.
4. "Risks for HIV Infection Among Persons Residing in Rural Areas and Small Cities—Selected Sites, Southern United States, 1995–1996." *Morbidity and Mortality Weekly Report* (11/20/98) Vol. 47, No. 45, P. 974.

Day 5: Learning

1. Centers for Disease Control & Prevention. "How long does it take for HIV to cause AIDS?" Fact Sheet. November, 1998.
2. Centers for Disease Control & Prevention. "How can I tell if I'm infected with HIV? What are the symptoms?" Fact Sheet. November, 1998.
3. Hecht, F., et al. "Use of laboratory tests and clinical symptoms for identification of primary HIV infection." AIDS 2002, 16:1119–1129.
4. Weber, R., et al. "Randomized, placebo-controlled trial of Chinese herb therapy for HIV-1-infected individuals." Journal of Acquired Immune Deficiency Syndromes 1999 Sep 1; 22(1):56–64.
5. Burack, J., et al. "Pilot randomized controlled trial of Chinese herbal treatment for HIV-associated symptoms." Journal of Acquired Immune Deficiency Syndromes and Human Retrovirology 1996 Aug 1; 12(4):386–93.
6. Lin, X., et al. "Clinical study on treatment of HIV infected persons based on viral load detection and CD4+T lymphocyte counting." Zhonghua Shi Yan He Lin Chuang Bing Du Xue Za Zhi 2002 Sep; 16 (3):211–4.

Day 6: Living

1. Kelly, J., et al. "Outcome of cognitive-behavioral and support group brief therapies for depressed, HIV-infected persons." American Journal of Psychiatry 1993 Nov; 150(11):1679–86.
2. Kelly, J., et al. "Factors associated with severity of depression and high-risk sexual behavior among persons diagnosed with human immunodeficiency virus (HIV) infection." Journal of Health Psychology 1993 May; 12(3):215–9.

Day 6: Learning

1. Normand, J., Vlahov, D., Moses, L. (eds.). Preventing HIV Transmission: The Role of Sterile Needles and Bleach. Washington, DC: National Academy Press, 1995.
2. Centers for Disease Control & Prevention. "Update: Syringe Exchange Programs—United States." Morbidity and Mortality Weekly Report 1998; 47:652–5.
3. Hagan, H., et al. "Volunteer bias in nonrandomized evaluations of the efficacy of needle-exchange programs." Journal of Urban Health 2000; 77:103–12.
4. Groseclose, S., et al. "Impact of increased legal access to needles and syringes on the practices of injecting-drug users and police officers—Connecticut, 1992–93." Journal of Acquired Immune Deficiency Syndromes and Human Retrovirology 1995; 10:82–9.
5. Academy for Educational Development. "Comprehensive approach: preventing bloodborne infections among injection drug users." Washington, DC: Academy for Educational Development, 2000. Available at http://www.cdc.gov/idu.

Day 7: Learning

1. Mellors, J., et al. "Plasma viral load and CD4+ lymphocytes as prognostic markers of HIV-1 infection." Annals of Internal Medicine 1997 Jun 15; 126(12):946–54. (Also found as Table V on page 39 of the August 13, 2001 issue of the "Guidelines for the Use of Antiretroviral Agents in HIV-infected Adults and Adolescents.")

Week 2: Living

1. Kitahata, M., et al. "Physicians' Experience with the Acquired Immunodeficiency Syndrome as a Factor in Patients' Survival." *New England Journal of Medicine*, Vol. 334:701–707 March 14, 1996, Number 11.
2. More, P., "Is Your Doctor in Financial Trouble?" *Thrive Magazine*, AIDS Healthcare Foundation. 2001.
3. Jecker, N., Braddock, C., "Managed Care." *Ethics in Medicine* 1998. University of Washington School of Medicine.
4. Herrick, D. "Would National Health Insurance Benefit Physicians?" Brief Analysis. No. 370, August 31, 2001, National Center for Policy Analysis.
5. Mechanic, D., McAlpine, D., Rosenthal, M. "Are Patients' Office Visits with Physicians Getting Shorter?" *New England Journal of Medicine* 2001 Jan. 18; Vol. 344, Num. 3:198–204.
6. Bartlett, J., Gallant, J. *2001–2002 Medical Management of HIV Infection*. Baltimore, MD: Johns Hopkins University Division of Infectious Diseases 2001.

Week 2: Learning

1. Smith, R. (Editor). *Encyclopedia of AIDS: A Social, Political, Cultural, and Scientific Record of the HIV Epidemic*. New York: Penguin, 2001.
2. U.S. Department of Health and Human Services. "Guidelines for the Use of Antiretroviral Agents in HIV-Infected Adults and Adolescents." February 04, 2002.

Week 3: Living

1. Canadian Psychiatric Association. *HIV & Psychiatry: A Training and Resource Manual*. Ottawa, Ontario: 2000.
2. Power, R., et al. "Self-disclosure of HIV serostatus in relation to depression and social support." Abstract. XIV International AIDS Conference, Barcelona, Spain, 2002.
3. Medved, W., et al. "Vulnerability of Men Who Have Sex With Men in Disclosing HIV-Positive Status to Sexual Partners and Significant Others: Need for Support and Assistance in Disclosure Decision-Making." XIV International AIDS Conference. Barcelona, Spain; July 7–12, 2002.
4. Logue, K., et al. "Coping with HIV+ Life: Experience of Recent Seroconverters." *The Canadian Journal of Infectious Diseases*, 9 (Suppl. A), March/April 1998.

Week 3: Learning

1. National Institute of Allergy and Infectious Diseases. "The Evidence That HIV Causes AIDS." Updated February, 2003. Available at:www.niaid.nih.gov/factsheets/evidhiv.htm.
2. Duesberg, P.D. *Inventing the AIDS Virus*. Washington: Regnery Publishing, 1996.

Week 4: Living

1. Cauffield, J. "The psychosocial aspects of complementary and alternative medicine." *Pharmacotherapy* 2000 Nov; 20(11):1289–94.
2. Project Inform. "Herbs, Supplements and HIV." Project Inform Fact Sheet. August 2000. For more information, http://www.projectinform.org.
3. Fairfield, K., et al. "Patterns of use, expenditures, and perceived efficacy of complementary and alternative therapies in HIV-infected patients." *Archives of Internal Medicine* 1998 Nov 9; 158(20):2257–64.
4. Burack, J., et al. "Pilot randomized controlled trial of Chinese herbal treatment for HIV-associated symptoms." *Journal of Acquired Immune Deficiency Syndromes and Human Retrovirology* 1996 Aug 1; 12(4):386–93.
5. Risa, K., et al. "Alternative therapy use in HIV-infected patients receiving highly active antiretroviral therapy." *International Journal of STD & AIDS* 2002 Oct; 13(10):706–13.
6. Ernst, E. "The risk-benefit profile of commonly used herbal therapies: Ginkgo, St. John's Wort, Ginseng, Echinacea, Saw Palmetto, and Kava." *Annals of Internal Medicine* 2002 Jan 1; 136(1):42–53.
7. U.S. Food and Drug Administration. "Kava-Containing Dietary Supplements May Be Associated with Severe Liver Injury." Consumer Advisory. March 25, 2002.
8. Piscitelli. S. "Indinavir Concentrations and St. John's Wort." *The Lancet*, Vol. 355, No. 9203, 12 February 2000.
9. Goldberg, B. *Alternative Medicine: The Definitive Guide.* Berkeley, California: Celestial Arts, 2002. (yoga: p. 465–473; massage: p. 503; meditation: p. 344–345).
10. Shekelle, P., et al. "Congruence Between Decisions to Initiate Chiropractic Spinal Manipulation for Low Back Pain and Appropriateness Criteria in North America." *Annals of Internal Medicine*, Vol. 129, 1998, pp. 9–17.
11. Shlay, J., et al. "Acupuncture and amitriptyline for pain due to HIV-related peripheral neuropathy: a randomized controlled trial. Terry Beirn Community Programs for Clinical Research on AIDS." *Journal of the American Medical Association* 1998 Nov 11; 280 (18):1590–5.

Week 4: Learning

1. The New Mexico AIDS InfoNet. "Fact Sheet 125: Viral Load Tests." New Mexico AIDS Education and Training Center, University of New Mexico Health Sciences Center, March 2003.
2. The New Mexico AIDS InfoNet. "Fact Sheet 124: T-Cell Tests." New Mexico AIDS Education and Training Center, University of New Mexico Health Sciences Center, November 2002.
3. U.S. Department of Health and Human Services. "Guidelines for the Use of Antiretroviral Agents in HIV-Infected Adults and Adolescents." February 04, 2002.

Month 2: Living

1. Page-Shafer, K., et al. "Risk of infection attributable to oral sex among men who have sex with men and in the population of men who have sex with men." *AIDS* 2002; 16, 17, 2350–2352.

2. Centers for Disease Control & Prevention. "How is HIV passed from one person to another?" Fact Sheet. November, 1998.
3. Page-Shafer, K., et al. "Risk of infection attributable to oral sex among men who have sex with men and in the population of men who have sex with men." *AIDS* 2002; 16, 17, 2350–2352.
4. Dillion, B., et al. "Primary HIV Infections Associated with Oral Transmission." Abstract #473, Poster Presentation. Seventh Conference on Retroviruses and Opportunistic Infections, San Francisco, January 30–February 2, 2000.
5. Trust, T. "Oral Sex Issues for Men With HIV." Briefing Sheet. September 2002.
6. Trust, T. "Oral Sex Issues for Women With HIV." Briefing Sheet. September 2002.
7. Trust, T. "Sexually Transmitted Infections: Issue for People with HIV." Briefing Sheet. September 2002.
8. Centers for Disease Control & Prevention. "Can I Get HIV from Having Vaginal Sex?" Fact Sheet. March 2003.
9. Canadian AIDS Society. *Safer Sex Guidelines, Healthy Sexuality and HIV: A Resource Guide for Educators and Counsellors.* Ottawa, 1994.
10. Jost, S., et al. "A Patient with HIV-1 Superinfection." *New England Journal of Medicine* 2002; 347:371.
11. Rhodes, T., Cusick, L. "Accounting for Unprotected Sex: Stories of Agency and Acceptability." *Social Science and Medicine* 2002 Jul; 55(2):211–26.
12. Mansergh, G., et al. "Barebacking in a Diverse Sample of Men Who Have Sex with Men." *AIDS* 2002 Mar 8; 16:653–659.
13. Castilla, J., et al. "Late Diagnosis of HIV Infection in the Era of Highly Active Antiretroviral Therapy: Consequences for AIDS Incidence." *AIDS* 2002 Sep 27; 16(14):1945–51.
14. Weller, S., Davis, K. "Condom Effectiveness in Reducing Heterosexual HIV Transmission." Cochrane Database of Systematic Reviews 2002; (1):CD003255.

Month 2: Learning

1. Fleming, D. T., et al. "Herpes Simplex Virus Type 2 in the United States, 1976 to 1994." *New England Journal of Medicine* 1997; 337:1105–1111.
2. Centers for Disease Control and Prevention. "Sexually Transmitted Diseases Treatment Guidelines." *Morbidity and Mortality Weekly Report* 2002; 51(RR–6).
3. Corey, L. "The Current Trend in Genital Herpes: Progress in Prevention." *Sex Trans Dis.* 1994; 21:S38–S44.
4. Langenberg, A., et al. "A Prospective Study of New Infections with Herpes Simplex Virus Type 1 and Type 2." *New England Journal of Medicine* 1999; 341:1432–1438.
5. Mertz, G. J., et al. "Risk Factors for the Transmission of Genital Herpes." *Annals of Internal Medicine* 1992; 116:197–202.
6. Wald, A., et al. "Reactivation of Genital Herpes Simplex Virus Type 2 Infection in Asymptomatic Seropositive Persons." *New England Journal of Medicine* 2000; 342:844–850.
7. Wald, A., Link, K. "Risk of Human Immunodeficiency Virus Infection in Herpes Simplex Virus Type-2 Seropositive Persons: A Meta-Analysis." *Journal of Infectious Diseases* 2002; 185:45–52.
8. Schacker, T. "The Role of HSV in the Transmission and Progression of HIV." *Herpes.* 2001; 8:46–49.

9. Schacker, T., et al. "Frequent Recovery of HIV-1 from Genital Herpes Simplex Virus Lesions in HIV-1 Infected Men." *Journal of the American Medical Association* 1998; 280:61–66.
10. Conant, M., et al. "Valaciclovir Versus Aciclovir for Herpes Simplex Virus Infection in HIV-Infected Individuals: Two Randomized Trials." *International Journal of STD & AIDS* 2002; 13:12–21.
11. Ho, G., et al. "Natural History of Cervicovaginal Papilloma Virus Infection in Young Women." *New England Journal of Medicine* 1998; 338:423–8.
12. Centers for Disease Control and Prevention. "Tracking the Hidden Epidemics 2000, Trends in STDs in the United States." 2001.
13. Bauer, H. M., et al. "Genital Human Papillomavirus Infection in Female University Students as Determined by a PCR-Based Method." *Journal of the American Medical Association* 1991; 265:472–477.
14. Palefsky, J. "Human Papillomavirus-associated Malignancies in HIV-positive Men and Women." *Current Opinion in Oncology* 1995; 7:437–441.
15. Minkoff, H., et al. "The Effect of Highly Active Antiretroviral Therapy on Cervical Cytologic Changes Associated with Oncogenic HPV Among HIV-infected Women." *AIDS* 2001; 15(16), pp. 2157–2164.
16. Pfister, H. "Relationship of Papillomaviruses to Anogenital Cancer." *Obstetrics and Gynecology Clinics of North America* 1987; 14:349–361.
17. Martins, C. "HPV-induced Anal Dysplasia: What Do We Know and What Can We Do About It?" *The Hopkins HIV Report*, May 2001.
18. National Institute of Allergy and Infectious Diseases. "Infection by Closely Related HIV Strains Possible." November 27, 2002, Press release. http://www.niaid.nih.gov.

Month 3: Living

1. National Institutes of Mental Health, "Depression." NIH Publication 2000; No. 00-3561.
2. Eller, L. "Effects of Cognitive-Behavioral Interventions on Quality of Life in Persons with HIV." *International Journal of Nursing Studies* 1999; 36:223–233.
3. May, T., et al. "Characteristics and Causes of Death Among HIV-infected Patients Who had a Good Immunovirologic Response under HAART: French National Survey (Mortalité 2000)." Abstract 913. Tenth Conference on Retroviruses and Opportunistic Infections 2003.
4. Kunches, L., et al. "Mental Health Diagnoses and Medications in HIV Patients Receiving Care in Publicly-funded Clinics." Poster. Ninth International AIDS Conference 2002.
5. Friedwald, V. *Ask the Doctor: Depression.* Kansas City, MI: Andrews McMeel Publishing 1998.
6. Bonacini, M., Puoti, M. "Hepatitis in Patients with Human Immunodeficiency Virus Infection." *Archives of Internal Medicine* 2000; 160:3365–3373.
7. Farber, E., et al. "Resilience Factors Associated with Adaptation to HIV Disease." *Psychosomatics* 2000; 41:140–146.
8. Sherbourne, C., et al. "Impact of Psychiatric Conditions on Health-Related Quality of Life in Persons with HIV Infection." *American Journal of Psychiatry* 2000;157:248–254.
9. Ling, S., et al. "Depression, Social Support, and Quality of Life in HIV Patients." Abstract 14343. Twelfth World AIDS Conference 1998.
10. Kelly, B., et al. "Suicidal Ideation, Suicide Attempts and HIV Infection." *Psychosomatics* 1998; 39:405–415.

Month 3: Learning

1. National Institutes of Mental Health. "Depression and HIV/AIDS." May 2002. NIH Publication No. 02-5005.
2. Stober, D., et al. "Depression and HIV Disease: Prevalence Correlates and Treatment." *Psychiatric Annals* 27(5): 372–377.
3. Risa, K., et al. "Determinants of Alternative Therapy Use in HIV Infected Patients Receiving HAART." Annual Meeting of the Association of Nurses in AIDS Care. October 2000.
4. Cabaj, R. "Management of Depression and Anxiety in HIV-Infected Patients." *Journal of the International Association of Physicians in AIDS Care.* June 1996.
5. Canadian Psychiatric Association. *HIV & Psychiatry: A Training and Resource Manual.* Ottawa, Ontario: 2000.

Month 4: Living

1. Turner, B., et al. "Effects of Drug Abuse and Mental Disorders on Use and Type of Antiretroviral Therapy in HIV-Infected Persons." *Journal of General Internal Medicine* 2001, Sep 16; (9):625–33.
2. "This Really Is Your Brain on Drugs, Scientist Explains." *RAND Review*, Fall 2000.
3. Bower, M., et al. "HIV-Related Lung Cancer in the Era of Highly Active Antiretroviral Therapy." *AIDS* 17:371–375, 2003.
4. Diaz, P., et al. "Increased Susceptibility to Pulmonary Emphysema Among HIV-Seropositive Smokers." *Annals of Internal Medicine* 2000 Mar 7; 132(5):369–72.
5. Samet, J. and others. "Alcohol Consumption and HIV Disease Progression: Are They Related?" *Alcoholism, Clinical and Experimental Research* 2003 May; 27(5): 862–867.
6. Abrams, D. I. and others. "Short-term Effects of Cannabinoids on HIV-1 Viral Load." Abstract and Late Breaker poster presentation LbPeB 7053 at the XIII International AIDS Conference. 2000 July 9–14; Durban, South Africa.
7. Beltrami, J., Park, M. "HIV Seroprevalence in Cocaine Users Treated at an Atlanta Drug Treatment Center." Georgia Epidemiology Report. 2000 June; Vol. 16, number 6.
8. Margolin, A., et al. "Cocaine, HIV, and Their Cardiovascular Effects: Is There a Role for ACE-Inhibitor Therapy?" *Drug and Alcohol Dependence* 2000 Dec 22; 61(1):35–45.

Month 4: Learning

1. U.S. Department of Health and Human Services, Public Health Service, Substance Abuse and Mental Health Services Administration, Center for Substance Abuse Treatment. "Substance Abuse Treatment for Persons with HIV/AIDS." Treatment Improvement Protocol Series 2000; no. 37.
2. National Institute on Drug Abuse, National Institutes of Health. "Principles of Drug Addiction Treatment: A Research-Based Guide." NIH Publication No. 00-4180, July 2000.
3. National Institute on Drug Abuse. "An Individual Drug Counseling Approach to Treat Cocaine Addiction." *Therapy Manuals for Drug Addiction.* U.S. Department of Health and Human Services 2001.

Month 5: Living

1. Sturm, R. "The Effects of Obesity, Smoking, and Problem Drinking on Chronic Medical Problems and Health Care Costs." *Health Affairs* 2002; 21(2):245–253.
2. Hodgsona, L., et al. "Wasting and Obesity in HIV Outpatients." *AIDS* 2001; 15:2341–2342.
3. Currier, J., et al. "Diabetes Mellitus in HIV-Infected Individuals." Poster Presentation, 2002. Ninth Conference on Retroviruses and Opportunistic Infections.
4. Fairfield, K., et al. "Patterns of Use, Expenditures, and Perceived Efficacy of Complementary and Alternative Therapies in HIV-infected Patients." *Archives of Internal Medicine* 1998 Nov 9; 158(20):2257–64.
5. Thompson, R. L., et al. "Dietary advice given by a dietitian versus other health professional or self-help resources to reduce blood cholesterol." *Cochrane Review* 2001; 1:CD001366.
6. Romanowski, A., Zullig, L. "Diet Wise, Pound Foolish: Promoted Diets for HIV." *AIDS Community Research Initiative of America Update*, Spring 2002. Vol. 11, No. 2.
7. Sutinen, J., et al. "Increased Fat Accumulation in the Liver in HIV-infected Patients with Antiretroviral Therapy-associated Lipodystrophy." *AIDS* 2002 Apr; 16(16): 2183–2193.
8. Hadigan, C., et al. "Modifiable Dietary Habits and Their Relation to Metabolic Abnormalities in Men and Women with Human Immunodeficiency Virus Infection and Fat Redistribution," *Clinical Infectious Diseases* 2001; 33:710–717.
9. Kosmiski, L. A., et al. "Fat Distribution and Metabolic Changes are Strongly Correlated and Energy Expenditure is Increased in the HIV Lipodystrophy Syndrome." *AIDS* 2001; 15:1993–2000.
10. Dube, M., et al. "Preliminary Guidelines for the Evaluation and Management of Dyslipidemia in Adults Infected with Human Immunodeficiency Virus and Receiving Antiretroviral Therapy: Recommendations of the Adult AIDS Clinical Trial Group Cardiovascular Disease Focus Group." *Clinical Infectious Diseases* 2000; 31:1216–1224.
11. BHIVA Writing Committee. "British HIV Association Guidelines for the Treatment of HIV-infected Adults with Antiretroviral Therapy." *HIV Medicine* 2001; 2:276–313.
12. Hooper, L. "Survey of UK Dietetic Departments: Diet in Secondary Prevention of Myocardial Infarction." *Journal of Human Nutrition and Dietetics* 2001; 14:307–318.
13. Hooper, L. "Dietary Fat Intake and Prevention of Cardiovascular Disease: Systematic Review." *British Medical Journal* 2001; 322:757–765.
14. Egger, M. "HAART and the Heart: Lipodystrophy and Cardiovascular Risk." *Physician's Research Network Notebook* 2001; 6:15–18.
15. Carr, A., et al. "A Syndrome of Peripheral Lipodystrophy, Hyperlipidaemia and Insulin Resistance in Patients Receiving HIV Protease Inhibitors." *AIDS* 1998; 12:F51–F58.
16. Wierzbicki, A. S. "Does Diet Have a Role in the Treatment of Hyperlipidaemia?" *International Journal of Clinical Practice* 2000; 54:72–73.
17. Moyle, G. J., et al. "Dietary Advice With or Without Pravastatin of Hypercholesterolaemia Associated with Protease Inhibitor Therapy." *AIDS* 2001; 15:1503–1508.
18. Tang, A. and others. "Weight Loss and Survival in HIV-Positive Patients in the Era of Highly Active Antiretroviral Therapy." *Journal of Acquired Immune Deficiency Syndromes* 2002; 31(2): 230–236.

Month 5: Learning

1. Samet, J., et al. "Trillion Virion Delay: Time From Testing Positive for HIV to Presentation for Primary Care." *Archives of Internal Medicine* 1998; 158:734–740.
2. Agency for Healthcare Research and Quality by the Research Triangle Institute-University of North Carolina at Chapel Hill Evidence-based Practice Center. "Management of Dental Patients Who Are HIV Positive." Evidence Report/Technology Assessment No. 37.
3. Project Inform. "Day One: After You've Tested Positive." Fact Sheet. January 1998.
4. Yeni , P. G., et al. "Antiretroviral Treatment for Adult HIV Infection in 2002." *Journal of the American Medical Association* 2002; 288:222.
5. Dybul, M., et al. "Antiretroviral Therapy for Adults and Adolescents." *Morbidity and Mortality Weekly Report* 2002; 51:RR–7:1.

Month 6: Living

1. Shapiro, M., et al. "The HIV Cost and Services Utilization Study." RAND and the Agency for Health Care Policy and Research, 1999.
2. Shapiro, M. F., et al. "Variations in the Care of HIV-Infected Adults in the United States." *Journal of the American Medical Association* 1999; 281:2305–2315.
3. National ADAP Monitoring Project. "Trends in Opportunistic Infection Drug Coverage and Spending." *Issue Brief*, February 2003.

Month 6: Learning

1. Americans With Disabilities Act of 1990. S. 933.
2. U.S. Equal Employment Opportunity Commission, U.S. Department of Justice Civil Rights Division. "Americans with Disabilities Act: Questions and Answers." http://www.usdoj.gov/crt/ada/qandaeng.htm.

Month 7: Living

1. Egger, M., et al. "Prognosis of HIV-1-infected Patients Starting Highly Active Antiretroviral Therapy: A Collaborative Analysis of Prospective Studies." *Lancet* 2002; 360:119.
2. Hadigan, C. and others. "Prediction of Coronary Heart Disease Risk in HIV-Infected Patients with Fat Redistribution." *Clinical Infectious Diseases* 2003 March; 36: 909–916.
3. Yeni, P., et al. "Antiretroviral Treatment for Adult HIV Infection in 2002." *Journal of the American Medical Association* 2002; 288:222.
4. Dybul, M., et al. "Antiretroviral Therapy for Adults and Adolescents." *Morbidity and Mortality Weekly Report* 2002; 51:RR-7:1.
5. U.S. Department of Health and Human Services. "Guidelines for the Use of Antiretroviral Agents in HIV-Infected Adults and Adolescents." February 04, 2002.
6. Robbins, G., et al. "Antiretroviral Strategies in Naïve HIV+ Subjects: Comparison of Sequential 3-drug Regimens." (ACTG 384). *NIAID News* 2002.

7. Little, S. J., et al. "Antiretroviral Drug Resistance Among Patients Recently Infected with HIV." *New England Journal of Medicine* 2002; 347:385.
8. Chambliss, P., et al. "Once daily HAART: A New Paradigm for HIV Treatment Success." Abstract MoPeB3293. XIV International AIDS Conference. July 7–12, 2002. Barcelona, Spain.

Month 8: Living

1. Sifakis, F., Hylton, J., Celentano, D. "Hepatitis B and Hepatitis C Infections Among Young Men Who Have Sex with Men." The Baltimore young men's survey. Abstract. Ninth Conference on Retroviruses and Opportunistic Infections.
2. Mohsen, A., et al. "Progression Rate of Liver Fibrosis in Human Immunodeficiency Virus and Hepatitis C Virus Co-infected Patients, UK Experience." Abstract MoOrB1057. XIV International AIDS Conference. Barcelona, Spain, July 7–12, 2002.

Month 8: Learning

1. Bartlett, J. "Top Papers of 2002." *The Johns Hopkins Report* 2003.
2. Consensus Developmental Panel: National Institutes of Health Consensus Developmental Conference Statement: Management of Hepatitis C. Available at http://www.consensus.nih.gov/cons/116/116cdc_intro.htm.

Month 9: Living

1. Carr, A., et al. "A Syndrome of Peripheral Lipodystrophy, Hyperlipidaemia and Insulin Resistance in Patients Receiving HIV Protease Inhibitors." *AIDS* 1998; 12:F51–F58.

Month 9: Learning

1. Schambelan, M., et al. "Management of Metabolic Complications Associated with Antiretroviral Therapy for HIV-1 Infection: Recommendations on an International AIDS Society-USA Panel," *Journal of Acquired Immune Deficiency Syndromes* 2002 Nov. 1; Vol. 31, 257–275.

Month 10: Living

1. Chesney, M. "Adherence to HAART Regimens." *AIDS Patient Care and STDS* 2003 Apr; 17(4): 169–177.
2. Ammassari, A., et al. "Determinants of Non-adherence in a Multi-center Cohort Study of Patients Previously Naïve to Antiretroviral Therapy." Program and Abstracts of the Fifth International Congress on Drug Therapy in HIV Infection, October 2000. Abstract 111.
3. Goujard, C., et al. "Factors Determining Adherence to HAART in a Cohort of 324 HIV-1-Infected Individuals." Program and Abstracts of the Fifth International Congress on Drug Therapy in HIV Infection, October 2000. Abstract 95.

Month 10: Learning

1. Clayton, J., et al. "Gender Differences in HIV Disease Progression." Program and Abstracts of the 13th International AIDS Conference, July 2000, Durban, South Africa. Abstract WePpD1344.

Month 11: Living

1. Cohen-Stuart, J., Wensing, A., and others. "Mechanisms Underlying Transient Relapses ("blips") of Plasma HIV RNA in Patients on HAART." Antiviral Therapy 2000; 5 (Supplement 3):107 and abstract 137 at the 4th International Workshop on HIV Drug Resistance and Treatment Strategies; June 12–16,2000; Sitges, Spain.
2. Havlir, D. and others. "Prevalence and Predictive Value of Intermittent Viremia in Patients with Viral Suppression." Antiviral Therapy 2000; 5 (Supplement 3):89 and abstract/oral presentation 112 at the 4th International Workshop on HIV Drug Resistance and Treatment Strategies; June 12–16, 2000; Sitges, Spain.

Month 11:Learning

1. Salama, C., Policar, M., Cervera, C. "Knowledge of Genotypic Resistance Mutations Among Providers of Care to Patients with Human Immunodeficiency Virus." Clinical Infectious Diseases 2003; 36:101–104.

Month 12: Living

1. Tuomala, R., et al. "Antiretroviral Therapy During Pregnancy and the Risk of Adverse Outcome." New England Journal of Medicine 2002; 346:1863.
2. Fundaro, C., et al. "Myelomeningocele in a Child with Intrauterine Exposure to Efavirenz." AIDS 2002; 16:299.
3. Minkoff, H. "Ethical Considerations in the Treatment of Infertility in Women with Human Immunodeficiency Virus Infection." The New England Journal of Medicine 2000 June 8; No. 23, Vol. 342:1748–1750.

Resources

National Hotlines
HIV and STDs

HIV/AIDS Information
Information about HIV/AIDS, TB,
STDs, referrals, references, workplace issues, and personal questions [CDC]
(800) 458-5231

HIV/AIDS and STD Hotline:
TTY-TDD: (800) 243-7889
Spanish: (800) 344-7432
English: (800) 342-2437

**Health Information for Sex
Workers:**
Hours 11-6, crisis intervention
(800) 676-4477

National Institutes of Health
Clinical trials information
(800) 243-7644

Legal

**Americans with Disabilities Act
Information and Assistance**
For questions about discrimination
(800) 514-0301

Federal Information Center
For questions about federal agencies,
programs, benefits, or services
TTY: (800) 326-2996
(800) 688-9889

Victims of Crime Hotline
Provides crisis intervention, assistance with the criminal justice
process, counseling, and support
groups
(800) 394-2255

Medicare Issues Hotline
Provides information about Medicare,
Medicaid, billing, benefits, coverage,
health plan choices, and claims
(800) 633-5227

Gay and Lesbian

Gay and Lesbian Hotline
General questions about gay and lesbian issues
(888) 843-4564

Pride Institute
Addiction treatment center for gay
and lesbian populations
(800) 547-7433

Hemophilia

Hemophilia and AIDS/HIV Network
(800) 424-2634

Youth

Child Abuse Hotline
Information about child abuse issues
(800) 422-4453

Runaway/Crisis Hotline for Teenagers
24-hour information for adolescents
(800) 621-4000

Youth Crisis, Runaway Hotline
Crisis information for youth 17 years and
younger
(800) 448-4663

Family

Domestic Violence Hotline
24-hour information, crisis intervention, and
referrals to local agencies
(800) 799-7233

Rape, Abuse, and Incest Hotline
(800) 656-4673

Pediatric and Family HIV Information
(800) 362-0071

Parents Anonymous Help Line
(800) 345-5044

Native Americans

Native American AIDS Information
(510) 444-2051

Women

Women with HIV Hotline
(800) 554-4876

Women's Health Information Center
(800) 994-9662

Rape, Abuse, and Incest Hotline
(800) 656-4673

Suicide

Suicide Hotline
For crisis calls
(800) 784-2433

HIV/AIDS Treatments

**HIV/AIDS Treatment Information
Service**
Information about HIV medications and clinical trials
(800) 448-0440

HIV Treatment Information
Information about HIV medications; calls
accepted from incarcerated individuals
(800) 822-7422

Veterans

VA Assistance Service
(800) 827-1000

Mental Health

Mental Health Association Help Line
Information on disorders and referrals to
mental health providers
(800) 969-6642

**National Mental Health Consumer
Self-Help Clearinghouse**
General inquiries
(800) 553-4539

Substance Abuse/ Addictions

Al-Anon and Alateen
Offers help and support for families and
friends of alcoholics
(888) 425-2666

Sexual Compulsives Anonymous
12-step program providing information about
local meetings
(800) 977-4325

Assisted Recovery
Offers a Naltrexone-based, non-12-step program of recovery from alcohol dependence
(800) 527-5344

Families Anonymous
12-step program for family members of people who may abuse drugs or alcohol
(800) 736-9805

Clearinghouse for Alcohol and Drug Information
(800) 729-6686

National Council on Alcoholism and Drug Dependence Hopeline
Information about counseling and treatment
(800) 622-2255

Drug and Alcohol Treatment Referral Service
Provides referrals to local organizations
(800) 662-4357

Cocaine Anonymous Referral Line
12-step program offering referrals to local meetings
(800) 347-8998

Substance Abuse and Mental Health Services Administration
(800) 789-2647

Pride Institute
Addiction treatment center for gay and lesbian populations
(800) 547-7433

Organizations Providing HIV/AIDS Services
UNITED STATES

ALABAMA
Alabama AIDS Hotline
In Alabama: (800) 228-0469
National: (334) 206-5364

AIDS Action Coalition of North Alabama
PO Box 871
Huntsville, AL 35804
(256) 536-4700, (800) 728-3603

AIDS Task Force of Alabama
PO Box 55703
Birmingham, AL 35255
Local: (205) 324-9822
Statewide Confidential Help Line:
(800) 592-2437

Mobile AIDS Support Services
2054 Dauphin St.
Mobile, AL 36606
(251) 471-5277

ALASKA
Alaska AIDS Hotline
In Alaska: (800) 478-2437
National: (907) 276-4880

Alaskan AIDS Assistance Association
1057 W. Fireweed, Suite 102
Anchorage, AK 99503
(907) 263-2050

Interior AIDS Association
710 Third Ave.
Fairbanks, AK 99707
(907) 452-4222

Shanti of Southeast Alaska
PO Box 22655
Juneau, AK 99801
(907) 463-5665, (800) 411-1331

ARIZONA
Arizona AIDS Hotline
In Arizona: (800) 334-1540
National: (602) 230-5819

AIDS Project Arizona
1427 N. 3rd St., Suite 125
Phoenix, AZ 85004
(602) 253-2437

Casa Gloriosa
3938 E. Grant Rd., #216
Tucson, AZ 85712
(520) 578-2749

Children With AIDS Project
PO Box 23778
Tempe AZ 85285-3778
(480) 774-9718

Southern Arizona AIDS Foundation
375 S. Euclid Ave.
Tucson, AZ 85719
(520) 628-7223, (800) 771-90F 4

Southwest Behavioral Health Services
Main Office (also locations throughout the state)
3707 North 7th St., #100
Phoenix, AZ 85014
(602) 265-8338

Tucson Interfaith HIV/AIDS Network
492 N. Alvernon Way
Tucson, AZ 85711
(520) 299-6647

ARKANSAS
Arkansas AIDS Hotline
In Arkansas: (800) 342-2437
National: (501) 661-2408

AIDS Service Society of Arkansas
518 East 9th St.
Little Rock, AR 72202
(501) 376-6299

Arkansas AIDS Foundation
PO Box 1208
Little Rock, AR 72203
(501) 376-6299, (800) 364-2437

Arkansas Children's Hospital AIDS Program
800 Marshall St., Slot 401
Little Rock, AR 72202
(501) 320-1406

Integrity
PO Box 55108
Little Rock, AR 72115
(501) 614-7200

Minority AIDS Network/Black Community Developers
4000 West 13th St.
Little Rock, AR 72204
(501) 663-9621

Regional AIDS Interfaith Network
800 S. Scott
PO Box 3776
Little Rock, AR 72203
(501) 376-6090, (800) 851-6301

Ryan White Center
510 McLean St.
Little Rock, AR 72203
(501) 376-6299

University of Arkansas for Medical Sciences (UAMS) AIDS Program
4301 W. Markham, Slot 639
Little Rock, AR 72205
(501) 686-7911, (501) 296-1682

AIDS Outreach of Arkansas
501 Maple St.
North Little Rock, AR 72114
(501) 372-5543, (888) 372-3703

CALIFORNIA (NORTHERN)
California HIV/AIDS Hotline
TDD: (888) 225-2437
In California: (800) 367-2437
In San Francisco and outside California:
(415) 863-2437

AIDS Community Research Consortium
1048 El Camino Real,
Redwood City, CA 94063-1633
(650) 364-6563

Asian & Pacific Islander Wellness Center
730 Polk St., 4th Floor
San Francisco, CA 94109
TTY: (415) 292-3410
(415) 292-3400

Diablo Valley AIDS Center
2490-G Arnold Industrial Way
Concord, California 94520-5328
(925) 686-3822

Genard AIDS Foundation
1630 North Main St., #102
Walnut Creek, CA 94596
(925) 943-2437

AIDS Resources, Information and Services of Santa Clara County
380 North 1st St., Suite #200
San Jose, CA 95112-4050
TDD: (408) 293-5836
(408) 293-2747

Multicultural AIDS Resource Center
390 4th St.
San Francisco, CA 94107
(415) 777-3229

AIDS Drug Assistance Program
995 Potrero Ave., Ward 86
San Francisco, CA 94110
(415) 206-3154

AIDS Emergency Fund
965 Mission St. #630
San Francisco, CA 94103
(415) 558-6999

AIDS Project of the East Bay
1755 Broadway, 2nd Floor
Oakland, CA 94612
(510) 663-7979

Black Coalition on AIDS
489 Clementina St.
San Francisco, CA 94103
(415) 615-9945

Center for AIDS Services
5720 Shattuck Ave.
Oakland, CA 94609
(510) 655-3435

Native American Health Center
56 Julian Ave.
San Francisco, CA 94110
(415) 621-8051

Project Inform
205 13th St., Suite 2001
San Francisco, CA 94103-2461
(415) 558-8669

Richmond Ermet AIDS Foundation
942 Divisadero St., Suite 201
San Francisco, CA 94115-4407
(415) 931-0317

San Francisco AIDS Foundation
995 Market St., #200
San Francisco, CA 94103
(415) 487-3000

UCSF AIDS Health Project
Client Services
1930 Market St.
San Francisco, CA 94102
(415) 476-3902

UCSF Community Consortium
3180 18th St., Suite 201
San Francisco, CA 94110
(415) 476-9554

Center for AIDS Research Education and Services
1500 21st St.
Sacramento, CA 95814
(916) 443-3299

Taylor Family Foundation
5555 Arroyo Rd.
Livermore, CA 94550
(925) 455-5118

CALIFORNIA (SOUTHERN)
California HIV/AIDS Hotline
TDD: (888) 225-2437
In California: (800) 367-2437

AIDS Healthcare Foundation
6255 W. Sunset Blvd., 21st Floor
Los Angeles, California 90028-7403
(323) 860-5200

L.A. Shanti
1616 N. La Brea Ave.
Los Angeles, CA 90028
(323) 962-8197

Los Angeles Free Clinic
8405 Beverly Blvd.
Los Angeles, CA 90048
(323) 653-1990

Los Angeles Free Clinic
Hollywood Center
6043 Hollywood Blvd.
Los Angeles, CA 90028
(323) 653-1990

Los Angeles Free Clinic
Hollywood Wilshire
Health Center
5205 Melrose Ave.
Los Angeles, CA 90038
(323) 653-1990

Being Alive
621 N. San Vicente Blvd.
West Hollywood, CA 90069
(310) 289-2551

Camp Pacific Heartland
5358 Cartwright Ave.
North Hollywood, CA 91601
(818) 753-6190

Correct HELP
PO Box 46276
West Hollywood, CA 90046
(323) 822-3830

AIDS Project Los Angeles
611 S. Kingsley Dr.
Los Angeles, CA 90010
(213) 201-1600

AIDS Project Los Angeles (West)
639 N. Fairfax Ave.
Los Angeles, CA 90036
(213) 201-1639

Asian Pacific AIDS Intervention Team
605 W. Olympic Blvd., #610
Los Angeles, CA 90015
(213) 553-1830

Bienestar Latino AIDS Project
4955 Sunset Blvd.
Los Angeles, CA 90027
(323) 660-9680

Bienestar Latino AIDS Project
5326 E. Beverly Blvd.
Los Angeles, CA 90022
(323) 727-7896

Bienestar Latino AIDS Project
1415 Hamlin St., #100
Van Nuys, CA 91405
(818) 908-3820

Bienestar Latino AIDS Project
180 E. Mission Blvd.
Pomona, CA 91766
(909) 397-7660

Los Angeles Jewish AIDS Services
PO Box 480241
Los Angeles, CA 90048
(323) 655-5330

Los Angeles Gay and Lesbian Center
1625 N. Schrader Blvd.
Los Angeles, CA 90028
(323) 993-7400

Minority AIDS Project
5149 Jefferson Blvd.
Los Angeles, CA 90016
(323) 936-4949

T.H.E. Clinic for Women
3860 W. Martin Luther King Blvd.
Los Angeles, CA 90008
(323) 295-6571

Minority AIDS Project
5149 W. Jefferson Blvd.
Los Angeles, CA 90016
(323) 936-4949

Watts Health Foundation
4116 E. Compton Blvd.
Compton, CA 90221
(310) 639-3068

Women Alive
1566 S. Burnside Ave.
Los Angeles, CA 90019
(323) 965-1564

Gay & Lesbian Community Center of Greater Long Beach
2017 E. 4th St.
Long Beach, CA 90803
(562) 434-4455

Whittier Rio Hondo AIDS Project
9200 Colima Rd., #104
Whittier, CA 90605
(562) 698-3850

AIDS Assistance Program
1276 N. Palm Canyon, Suite #108
Palm Springs, CA 92262
(760) 325-8481

Desert AIDS Project
PO Box 2890
Palm Springs, CA 92263-2890
(760) 323-2118, (866) 331-3344

Being Alive San Diego
Centre Street Office
4070 Centre St.
San Diego, CA 92103
(619) 291-1400

Being Alive San Diego
North County Office
804 Pier View Way
Oceanside, CA 92054
(760) 439-6908

HIV Consumer Council
Office of Aids Coordination
Health and Human Services Agency
PO Box 85524 MS P501-C
San Diego, CA 92186

POZabilities
San Diego, CA
(619) 908-6479

Asian Pacific Islander Community AIDS Project
4776 El Cajon Blvd., Suite 204
San Diego, CA 92115
(619) 229-2822

Sunburst Projects
5350 Commerce Blvd., Suite I
Rohnert Park, CA 94928
(707) 588-9477

COLORADO

Colorado AIDS Hotline
Denver only: (303) 782-5186
In Colorado: (800) 252-2437

Boulder County AIDS Project
2118 14th St.
Boulder, CO 80302
(303) 444-6121, Spanish: (303) 444-7181

Northern Colorado AIDS Project
400 Remington St., Suite 100
PO Box 182
Fort Collins, CO 80524
(970) 484-4469

Southern Colorado AIDS Project
1301 South Eighth St., Suite 200
Colorado Springs, CO 80906
(719) 578-9092, (800) 241-5468

CONNECTICUT

AIDS Project Hartford
110 Bartholomew Ave.
Hartford, CT 06106-2241
TTY: (860) 951-4791
(860) 951-4833

Connecticut AIDS Residence Coalition
56 Arbor St.
Hartford, CT 06106
(860) 231-8212

Mid-Fairfield AIDS Project
16 River St.
Norwalk, CT 06580-3104
(203) 855-9535

Northwestern Connecticut AIDS Project
100 Migeon Ave.
Torrington, CT 06790
Local: (860) 482-1596
(800) 381-2437

DELAWARE

Delaware AIDS Hotline
In Delaware: (800) 422-0429
National: (302) 652-6776

AIDS Delaware
New Castle County Office
100 West 10th St., Suite 315
Wilmington, DE 19801
(302) 652-6776

AIDS Delaware
Kent & Sussex County Office
706 Rehoboth Ave., Suite 1
Rehoboth Beach, DE 19971
(302) 226-5350

Delaware HIV Consortium
100 West 10th St., Suite 415
Wilmington, DE 19801
(302) 654-5471

Sussex County AIDS Committee
107 South St.
PO Box 712
Rehoboth Beach, DE 19971
(302) 644-1090

DISTRICT OF COLUMBIA

District of Columbia AIDS Information Line
(202) 332-2437
In metro DC and VA: (800) 322-7432

AIDS Alliance for Children, Youth & Families
1600 K St. NW, Suite 200
Washington, DC 20006
Local: (202) 785-3564
(888) 917-2437

Food & Friends
58 L St. SE
Washington, DC 20003
TDD:(202) 554-2944
(202) 488-8278

Metro TeenAIDS
PO Box 15577
Washington, DC 20003-5577
(202) 543-9355

P.L.Active
1772 Church St. NW
Washington, DC 20009

National Minority AIDS Council
1931 13th St. NW
Washington, DC 20009
(202) 483-6622

Washington AIDS International Foundation
3224 16th St. NW
Washington, DC 20010
(202) 745-0111

Whitman-Walker Clinic
1407 S St. NW
Washington, DC 20009
TDD: (202) 939-1578
Spanish: (202) 328-0697
Gay/Lesbian Hotline: (202) 833-3234
AIDS Info Line: (877) 939-2437
24-Hour Line: (202) 365-5225
(202) 797-3500

YouthAIDS
1120 19th St., Suite 600
Washington, DC 20036
(202) 785-0072

FLORIDA
Florida AIDS Hotline
In Florida, in English: (800) 352-AIDS
In Haitian Creole: (800) 243-7101
In Spanish: (800) 545-SIDA
TTY: (888) 503-7118
National: (850) 681-9131

Care Resource
1320 South Dixie Highway, Suite 485
Coral Gables, FL 33146
(305) 667-9296

Florida AIDS Action
PO Box 16705
Tampa, FL 33687-6705
(813) 232-5886
Toll Free in Florida: (800) 779-4898

Florida AIDS Action
Miami Office
PMB 151
12864 Biscayne Blvd.
North Miami, FL 33181-2007
(305) 891-3666

Florida AIDS Action
Tallahassee Office
1375 Cross Creek Circle
Tallahassee, FL 32301
(850) 656-7760, Ext. 300

Joe Logsdon Foundation
2496 Kirkwood Ave.
Naples, FL 34112
(239) 417-8400

League Against AIDS
3050 Biscayne Blvd., Suite 503
Miami, FL 33137
(305) 576-1000

North Central Florida AIDS Network
3615 S.W. 13th St., Suites 3 & 4
Gainesville, FL 32608
(352) 372-4370, (800) 824-6745

Palm Beach County HIV Care Council
4152 West Blue Heron Blvd.
Riviera Beach, FL 33404
(561) 844-4430, Ext. 14

People With AIDS Coalition of Broward
2302 NE 7th Ave.
Ft. Lauderdale, FL 33305
(954) 565-9119

South Beach AIDS Project
1521 Alton Rd., #403
Miami Beach, FL 33139
(305) 532-1033

Tampa AIDS Network
North Tampa Office
7402 North 56th St.
Bldgs. 100 & 200
(813) 914-8888

Tampa AIDS Network
South Tampa Office
2901 Swann Ave., Suite 107
(813) 879-4700

GEORGIA
Georgia AIDS Information Line
In Georgia: (800) 551-2728
National: (404) 876-9944

AID Atlanta
1438 W. Peachtree St. NW, Suite 100
Atlanta, GA 30309-2955
TTY/Voice: (404) 870-7773
(404) 870-7700

AIDS Research Consortium of Atlanta
131 Ponce de Leon Ave. NE, Suite 130
Atlanta, GA 30308
(404) 872-2873

AIDS Survival Project
159 Ralph McGill Blvd., Suite 500
Atlanta, GA 30308
TTY: (404) 524-0464
(404) 874-7926

Safe Haven
Referrals available by calling:
(229) 225-3997

HAWAII
Hawaii STD/AIDS Hotlines
In Hawaii: (800) 321-1555
National: (808) 922-1313

Maui AIDS Foundation
1935 Main St., Suite 101
PO Box 858
Wailuku, Maui HI 96793
(808) 242-4900

Maui AIDS Foundation
Moloka'i Office
PO Box 341
Kaunakakai, HI 96748
(808) 553-9086

Maui AIDS Foundation
Hana Office
PO Box 875
Hana, HI 96713
(808) 248-7801

Maui AIDS Foundation
Lana'i Office
PO Box 1329
Lana'i City, HI 96763
(808) 565-6722

IDAHO
Idaho AIDS Foundation Hotline
In Idaho: (800) 926-2588
National: (208) 321-2777

North Idaho AIDS Coalition
410 Sherman Ave., Suite 215
Coeur d'Alene, ID 83814
(208) 665-1448

South Central Idaho AIDS Coalition
213 East Ave. D
Jerome, ID 83338
(208) 734-5900, ext. 269

ILLINOIS
In Illinois
TTY/TDD: (800) 782-0423
National: (217) 785-7165

AIDS Care
315 W. Barry
Chicago, IL 60657
(773) 935-4663

AIDS Legal Council of Chicago
188 West Randolph St., Suite 2400
Chicago, IL 60601-3005
(312) 427-8990

Bethany Place
821 West A St.
Belleville, IL 62220
(618) 234-0291

Better Existence With HIV
(847) 475-2115

Central Illinois Friends of PWA
415 St. Marks Ct., Suite 504
Peoria, IL 61603
(309) 671-2144

Coalition for Positive Sexuality
Broadway PMB#191
Chicago, IL 60613
(773) 604-1654

HIV Coalition
990 Criss Circle
Elk Grove Village, IL 60007
(847) 228-5200

Howard Brown Health Center
4025 N. Sheridan Rd.
Chicago, IL 60613
(773) 388-1600

Test Positive Aware Network
5537 N. Broadway St.
Chicago, IL 60640-1405
(773) 989-9400

Jewish AIDS Network–Chicago
(773) 275-2626

Open Door Clinic
164 Division St., Suite #607
Elgin, IL 60120
(847) 695-1093

Open Door Clinic
Aurora Office
157 S. Lincoln Ave., Room K
Aurora, IL 60505
(630) 264-1819

INDIANA
Indiana Community AIDS Action Network
3951 North Meridian St., Suite 200
Indianapolis, IN 46208
(317) 920-3190, Ext. 307

AIDS Task Force Southeast Central Indiana
1401 Chester Blvd.
Jenkins Hall, 5th Floor
Richmond, IN 47374
(765) 983-3425, Ext. 0

Damien Center
1350 N. Pennsylvania
Indianapolis, IN 46202
(317) 632-0123, (800) 213-1163

Harm Reduction Institute
133 West Market St., Suite 197
Indianapolis, IN 46204
(317) 974-1940

Prevention Point of Indiana
133 West Market St., Suite 201
Indianapolis, IN 46204
(317) 780-0001

Project AIDS Lafayette
1306 E. Main. St.
Crawfordsville, IN 47933
(317) 361-5818

IOWA

Iowa AIDS Hotline
In Iowa: (800) 445-2437
National: (515) 244-6700

Dubuque Regional AIDS Coalition
1454 Iowa St.
Dubuque, IA 52001
(563) 589-4181

Rapids AIDS Project
American Red Cross
3601 42nd St. NE
Cedar Rapids, IA 52402
(319) 393-9579

KANSAS

Douglas County AIDS Project
United Way Center for Human Resources
2518 Ridge Ct., Room 244
Lawrence, KS 66046
(785) 843-0040

Aids Resource Network of Southeast Kansas
(800) 738-2437

KENTUCKY

AIDS Services Center Coalition, Inc.
(502) 574-5490

AIDS Interfaith Ministries of Kentuckiana
(502) 574-6085, (502) 574-6086

Family & Children's Counseling Centers
(502) 583-1741

HIV/AIDS Legal Project of the Legal Aid Society
(502) 574-8199

House of Ruth
(502) 587-5080

Jefferson County Health Department
(502) 574-5600

Jefferson County Health Department Specialty Clinic
(502) 574-6699

Louisville Youth Group
(502) 894-9787

Louisville/Jefferson County Minority AIDS Program
(502) 585-4733
Offices in Louisville, Lexington, Hopkinsville, and Bowling Green

Volunteers of America STOP Program
(502) 635-1361

WINGS Clinic
(502) 852-2523

AIDS Volunteers
263 N. Limestone St.
Lexington, KY 40507
(859) 225-3000

LOUISIANA

Louisiana AIDS Hotline
In Louisiana: (800) 992-4379
In Louisiana: (504) 944-2437
In Louisiana TDD: (504) 944-2492
National: (785) 296-6036

NO/AIDS Task Force
2601 Tulane Ave., Suite 500
New Orleans, LA 70119
(504) 821-2601

Food for Friends
2533 Columbus St.
New Orleans, LA 70119
(504) 944-6028

Community Awareness Network
507 Frenchmen St.
New Orleans, LA 70116
(504) 945-4000

Friends for Life
660 North Foster Dr., Building C-100
Baton Rouge, LA 70806
(225) 923-2277

MAINE
The Maine AIDS Alliance
39 Green St.
Augusta, ME 04330
(207) 621-2924

MARYLAND
Maryland AIDS Hotline
In Maryland (Bilingual) (800) 638-6252
In Metro DC & VA: (800) 322-7432
Hispanic AIDS Hotline: (301) 949-0945
Baltimore only TTY area: (410) 333-2437
National: (410) 767-5013

Deaf AIDS Project (Baltimore)
Family Service Foundation
2310 North Charles St.
Baltimore, MD 21218
TTY: 410-889-8077
MD Relay: 711
(888) 840-3266, (410) 889-8040, Ext. 27

Food & Friends (serving Maryland)
58 L St. SE
Washington, DC 20003
TDD: (202) 554-2944
(202) 488-8278

National Association for Victims of Transfusion-Acquired AIDS
8721 Burdette Rd.
Bethesda, MD 20817
(301) 365-8750

Chase Brexton Health Services
Baltimore City
1001 Cathedral St.
Baltimore, MD 21201
(410) 837-2050

Chase Brexton Health Services
Baltimore County
4000 Old Court Rd., Suite 203
Baltimore, MD 21208
(410) 486-5991

Health Education Resource Organization
Maryland Community Resource Center
1734 Maryland Ave.
Baltimore, MD 21201
(410) 685-1180

MASSACHUSETTS
Massachusetts AIDS Hotline
In Massachusetts: (800) 235-2331
National: (617) 536-7733
TTY/TDD: (617) 437-1672
Youth Only AIDS Line toll-free at (800) 788-1234,
TTY: (617) 450-1427

AIDS Action Committee of Massachusetts
131 Clarendon St.
Boston, MA 02116
TTY: (617) 437-1394
(617) 437-6200; (800) 235-2331

AIDS Project Worcester
Worcester Office
85 Green St.
Worcester, MA 01604
(508) 755-3773

South County Office
39 Elm St.
Southbridge MA 01550
(508) 765-2670, (508) 765-3812

North County Office
14 Monument Sq., Suite 101D
Leominster MA 01453
(978) 466-6868

Boston Living Center
29 Stanhope St.
Boston, MA 02116
(617) 236-1012

Common Sensitivity
1 Main St.
Leominster, MA 01453-5501
(978) 840-4673, (888) 840-4673

Community Research Initiative of New England
23 Miner St.
Boston, MA 02215-3318
TTY: (617) 778-5460
(617) 778-5454, (888) 253-2712

Community Research Initiative of New England
Springfield Office
780 Chestnut St., Suite 30
Springfield, MA 01107
(413) 734-2264, (888) 469-6577

North Shore AIDS Health Project
67 Middle St.
Gloucester, MA 01930
(978) 283-0101

Positive Directions in Boston
140 Clarendon St., Suite 805
Boston, MA 02116
(617) 262-3456

Search for a Cure
34 Edgerly Rd., #1
Boston, MA 02115
(617) 536-2474

TeenAIDS PeerCorps
PO Box 146727
Boston, MA 02114
(978) 665-9383

MICHIGAN

Michigan AIDS Hotline
In Michigan: (800) 872-2437
TTY/TDD: (800) 332-0849
Spanish: (800) 826-SIDA
Teen Line: (800) 750-TEEN
Health Care Workers: (800) 522-0399
National: (313) 446-9800

AIDS Care Network (Grand Rapids)
207 Fulton East, 4th Floor
Grand Rapids, MI 49503
(616) 774-2042

AIDS Partnership Michigan
2751 E. Jefferson, Suite 301
Detroit, MI 48207
(313) 446-9800

B.A.S.I.S.
Serving Bay, Saginaw, Midland, Huron, Sani-
lac and Tuscola Counties
515 Adams St.
Bay City, MI 48708
(517) 894-2991, (800) 727-2527

Community AIDS Resource & Education Services
629 Pioneer St.,
Kalamazoo, MI 49008-1801
(616) 381-2437, (800) 944-2437

Corner Health Center
47 N. Huron St.
Ypsilanti, MI 48197
(734) 484-3600

Friends Alliance
4513 East 9 Mile Rd.
Warren, MI 48091-2596
(586) 759-5940, (800) 350-7927

HIV/AIDS Resource Center
3075 Clark Rd., Suite 203
Ypsilanti, MI 48197
(734) 572-9355, (800) 578-2300

HIV/AIDS Wellness Networks Grand Traverse Area
516 East Eighth St.
Traverse City MI 49684
(231) 933-0279

Lansing Area AIDS Network
913 West Holmes, Suite 115
Lansing, MI 48910
(517) 394-3560

AIDS Interfaith Network
2751 East Jefferson Ave., Suite 301
Detroit, MI 48207
(313) 446-9800

AIDS Law Project
(313) 962-0466, Ext. 348

AIDS Support Group/Tri- Cities
PO Box 6361
Saginaw, MI 48603
(517) 758-3877

Alternatives For Girls
1950 Trumbull
Detroit, MI 48216
(313) 496-0938

American Civil Liberties Union
1249 Washington Blvd., Suite 2910
Detroit, MI 48226-1822
(313) 961-4662

Bay Area Social Intervention Services
904 6th St.
Bay City, MI 48708-6527
(517) 894-2991

Black Family Development
15231 West McNichols
Detroit, MI 48235
(313) 272-3500

Children's Immune Disorder
16888 Greenfield
Detroit, MI 48235-3707
(313) 837-7800

Community Health Awareness Group
3028 East Grand Blvd.
Detroit, MI 48202
(313) 872-2424

Community Recover Services
711 N. Saginaw, Suite 323
Flint, MI 48503
(810) 238-2068

Detroit American Indian Health and Family Services
4880 Lawndale
Detroit, MI 48210
(313) 846-3781

Detroit Central City Community Mental Health
10 Peterburg, Suite 230
Detroit, MI 48201
(313) 831-3160

Hemophilia Foundation of Michigan
905 W. Eisenhower, #107
Ann Arbor, MI 48103
(734) 332-4226

Hispanics Against AIDS
730 Grandville
Grand Rapids, MI 49503
(616) 742-0200

HIV/AIDS Network and Direct Services
PO Box 533
Petoskey, MI 49770
(231) 526-9213, (888) 526-9213

HIV/AIDS Services
345 State SE
Grand Rapids, MI 49503
(616) 456-9063, (888) 619-9900

HIV/AIDS Wellness Networks
516 E. 8th St., PO Box 1632
Traverse City, MI 49685
(231) 933-0279

Lansing Area AIDS Network
4660 Hagadorn Rd., Suite 510
East Lansing, MI 48823
(517) 351-4534

Latino Family Services
3815 West Fort St.
Detroit, MI 48209
(313) 841-7380

Muskegon Area AIDS Resource Services
500 W. Western, Suite 750
Muskegon, MI 49440
Within 231 Area Code: (231) 722-2437
(888) 995-6399

Neighborhood Services Department
Drug Treatment Program
5031 Grandy Ave.
Detroit, MI 48211
(313) 267-6718

Tribal Health and Human Services
2864 Ashmun St.
Sault Ste. Marie, MI 49783
(906) 632-5265

University of Michigan HIV/AIDS Treatment Program
Department of Internal Medicine
3120 Taubman Center
Ann Arbor, MI 48109-0378
(734) 763-9227

Muskegon Area AIDS Resource Services
500 W. Western Ave., Suite 750
Muskegon, MI 49440
(231) 722-2437

MINNESOTA
Minnesota AIDS Line
National: (612) 373-2437
In Minnesota: (800) 248-2437

The Aliveness Project
730 East 38th St.
Minneapolis, MN 55407
(612) 822-7946

Delaware Street Clinic
Building Address:
Room G254
Mayo Building
420 Delaware St. SE
Box 88
Mail:
Mayo Building
420 Delaware St. SE
Minneapolis, MN 55455
(612) 625-4680,
   (800) 688-5252, Ext. 5-4680

Minnesota AIDS Project
1400 Park Ave. South
Minneapolis, MN 55404
(612) 341-2060

Rural AIDS Action Network
3112 Hennepin Ave.
Minneapolis, MN 55408
(612) 827-0862, (800) 966-9735

Youth and AIDS Projects
University of Minnesota
428 Oak Grove St.
Minneapolis, MN 55403
(612) 627-6820

MISSISSIPPI

Mississippi AIDS Hotline
In Mississippi: (800) 826-2961
National: (601) 576-7723

Coastal Family Health Services
683 Division St.
Biloxi, MS 39533
(228) 374-4991

South Mississippi AIDS Task Force
221 Rue Petit Bois, Building D
PO Box 8009
Biloxi, MS 39535
(228) 385-1214, (800) 826-2961

DePorres Health Center
411 Poplar St.
Marks, MS 38646
(228) 385-1214, (601) 326-9232

G. A. Carmichael Family Health Center
PO Box 588
1668 West Peace St.
Canton, MS 39046
(601) 859-5213

Aaron E. Henry Community Health Center
PO Box 1216
1040 DeSoto Ave.
Clarksdale, MS 38614
(601) 624-4292

Jefferson Comprehensive Health Center
PO Box 98
225 Community Dr.
Fayette, MS 39069
(601) 786-3475

Magnolia Medical Clinic
1411 Strong Ave.
Greenwood, MS 38930
(663) 459-1277

Southeast Mississippi Rural Health Initiative
PO Box 1729
Hattiesburg, MS 39403
(601) 545-8700

Building Bridges in Jackson
PO Box 55433
Jackson, MS 39296
(601) 922-0100

Catholic Charities
PO Box 2248
530 George St.
Jackson, MS 39225
(601) 355-8634

Central Mississippi Circle of Care
350 W. Woodrow Wilson, Suite 751
Jackson, MS 39213
(601) 815-1323

Episcopal AIDS Committee
PO Box 55803
Jackson, MS 39296
(601) 936-6780

Jackson State University
National Alumni AIDS Prevention
PO Box 18890
1400 J. R. Lynch
Jackson, MS 39217
(601) 968-2519

Mississippi State Department of Health
HIV/AIDS Prevention
570 E. Woodrow Wilson, Suite 350
PO Box 1700
Jackson, MS 39215
(601) 576-7723

Project Connect AIDS Service Organization
350 W. Woodrow Wilson, Suite 3210
Jackson, MS 39213
(601) 981-1700

University of Mississippi Medical Center
Infectious Diseases Department
2500 North State St.
Jackson, MS 39216
(601) 984-5552

University of Mississippi Pediatric AIDS
2500 North State St.
Jackson, MS 39216
(601) 984-5206

VA Medical Center
PWA Support Group
1500 Woodrow Wilson Dr.
Jackson, MS 39216
(601) 362-4471, Ext. 1776

Greater Meridian Health Clinic
2701 Davis St.
Meridian, MS 39301
(601) 693-0118

Sharp Family Care Center
101 Hospital Dr.
Tylertown, MS 39667
(601) 876-4926

Sacred Heart Southern Mission
6144 Highway 61 North, Box 5
Walls, MS 38680
(662) 781-2295

MISSOURI

Missouri AIDS Information Line
National: (800) 533-2437

AIDS Foundation of St. Louis
5615 Pershing Ave., Suite 11
St. Louis, MO 63112
(314) 367-7273

MONTANA

Montana AIDS PROGRAM
In Montana: (800) 233-6668
National: (406) 444-3565
Eastern Montana AIDS Hotline:
(800) 675-2437
Western Montana AIDS Hotline:
(800) 663-9002

Butte AIDS Support Services
PO Box 382
Butte, MT 59703
(406) 496-6125

Falls AIDS Network
2611 10th Ave. South
PO Box 220
Great Falls, MT 59405
(406) 771-8861

Flathead AIDS Council
723 5th Ave. East
Kalispell, MT 59901
(406) 752-5500

Lewis and Clark AIDS Project
PO Box 832
Helena, MT 59624
(406) 449-1357

Mission Valley AIDS Council
802 Main St.
Polson, MT 59860
(406) 883-7314

Missoula AIDS Council
415 N. Higgins, Suite 109
Missoula, MT 59802
(406) 543-4770

Montana Migrant Health Project
3318 3rd Ave. N 100
Billings, MT 59101-1900
(406) 248-3149

PRIDE!
PO Box 775
Helena, MT 59624
(800) 610-9322, (406) 442-9322

Ravalli County HIV/AIDS Education and Prevention Council
PO Box 190
Stevensville, MT 59870
(406) 777-3646

AIDS Network of Southern Montana
321 East Main St., Suite 409
Bozeman, MT 59715
(406) 582-1110

Valley County AIDS Task Force
501 Court House Sq., Box 11
Glasgow, MT 59230
(406) 228-8221, Ext. 61

Wheatland County AIDS Task Force
Wheatland Community Hospital
Harlowton, MT 59036
(406) 632-4351

Yellowstone AIDS Project
208 N. 29th St., Suite 230
Billings, MT 59103
(406) 245-2029

NEBRASKA
Nebraska AIDS Hotline
National: (800) 782-2437

Nebraska AIDS Project
Omaha & Watanabe Wellness Center
139 South 40th St.
Omaha, NE 68131
(402) 552-9260

Nebraska AIDS Project
Lincoln Office
220 South 17th St.
Lincoln, NE 68508
(402) 476-7000

Nebraska AIDS Project
Norfolk Office
304 North 5th St., Suite C
Norfolk, NE 68701
(402) 370-3300

Nebraska AIDS Project
Kearney Office
3423 Second Ave.
Kearny, NE 68847
(308) 865-5610

Nebraska AIDS Project
Scottsbluff Office
4500 Ave. I, PO Box 1500
Scottsbluff, NE 69361
(308) 635-3807

NEVADA
Nevada AIDS Information Line
In Nevada: (800) 842-2437

Aid for AIDS of Nevada
2300 South Rancho Dr., Suite 211
Las Vegas, NV 89102
(702) 382-2326

Golden Rainbow
1700 East Desert Inn Rd., Suite #311
Las Vegas, NV 89109
(702) 384-2899

Northern Nevada H.O.P.E.S
PO Box 6420
Reno, NV 89513
(775) 786-4673

NEW HAMPSHIRE
New Hampshire AIDS Hotline
In New Hampshire: (800) 752-2437
National: (603) 271-4502

New Hampshire/Vermont HIV Information Network
PO Box 882
Bellows Falls, VT 05101
(888) 338-8796

NEW JERSEY
New Jersey AIDS Hotline
In New Jersey: (800) 624-2377 (24 hrs., 7 days)
TTY/TDD: (201) 926-8008
National: (973) 926-7443

AIDS Coalition of Southern New Jersey
100 Essex Ave., Suite 300
Bellmawr, NJ 08031
(856) 933-9500

Hyacinth AIDS Foundation
78 New St., Second Floor
New Brunswick, NJ 08901
(732) 246-0204
Hotline: (800) 433-0254 (available in NJ only, TDD accessible); outside of NJ, call (732) 246-0204

National Pediatric & Family HIV Resource Center
University of Medicine & Dentistry of
   New Jersey
30 Bergen St.— ADMC #4
Newark, NJ 07103
(973) 972-0410, (800) 362-0071

Buddies of New Jersey
Franklin A. Smith Resource Center
149 Hudson St.
Hackensack NJ 07601
(201) 489-2900, (800) 508-7577

South Jersey AIDS Alliance
19 Gordon's Alley
Atlantic City, NJ 08401
(609) 347-1085

Good Shepard Community Services
1576 Palisade Ave.
Ft. Lee, NJ 07024

Mercer County AIDS Consortium
447 Bellevue Ave.
Trenton, NJ 08618
(609) 278-9555

Middlesex County HIV Resource Center
275 Hobart St.
Perth Amboy, NJ 08861

Monmouth-Ocean HIV Care Consortium
625 Bangs Ave.
Asbury Park, NJ 07712
(732) 505-5122

Passaic County AIDS Resource Center
100 Hamilton Plaza, Room 707
Paterson, NJ 07505
(973) 742-6742

Somerset-Hunterdon HIV Care Consortium
95 Veteran's Memorial Dr.
Somerville, NJ 07505
(908) 704-9641

South Jersey Council on AIDS
120 White Horse Pike, Suite 110
Haddon Heights, NJ 08035
(609) 547-6600

HIV Care Consortium/Resource Center
16 South Ohio Ave.
Atlantic City, NJ 08035
(609) 441-8181

Union County HIV Consortium
80 West Grand St., Lower Level
Elizabeth, NJ 07202
(908) 352-7700

NEW MEXICO
New Mexico AIDS Hotline
In New Mexico: (800) 545-2437
National: (505) 476-3612

Camino de Vida
2805 Doral Ct.
PO Drawer 2827
Las Cruces, New Mexico 88004
(505) 532-0202, (800) 687-0850

HIV/AIDS Law Panel New Mexico
(800) 982-2021

Southwest Comprehensive AIDS-Care Center
649 Harkle Rd., Suite E
Santa Fe, New Mexico 87505
(505) 989-8200, (888) 320-8200

HIV/AIDS Support
(505) 521-4387

NEW YORK
New York State HIV counseling hotline: (800) 872-2777
National: (716) 845-3170
New York State information hotline:
   (800) 541-2437
New York State Spanish hotline:
   (800) 233-SIDA

Women and AIDS Resources Network
135 West 4th St.
New York, NY 10012
(212) 475-6713

AIDS Treatment Data Network
611 Broadway, Suite 613
New York, NY 10012
(800) 734-7104

Gay Men's Health Crisis
119 West 24th St.
New York, NY 10011
(212) 807-6655

Long Island Association for AIDS Care
755 Park Ave. (Broadway)
Huntington, New York 11743
(516) 385-2437

Task Force on AIDS of New York State
Psychological Association
(212) 459-4167

Hispanic AIDS Forum
Manhattan Office
184 Fifth Ave., Floor 7
New York, NY 10010
(212) 741-9797

Hispanic AIDS Forum
Queens Office
74-09 37 Ave., Suite 305
Jackson Heights, NY 11372
(718) 803-2766

Hispanic AIDS Forum
Bronx Office
886 Westchester Ave.
Bronx, NY 10459
(718) 328-4188

AIDS Council of Northeastern New York
Albany South End Office
88 Fourth Ave.
Albany, NY 12202
(518) 434-4686, (800) 660-6886

AIDS Council of Northeastern New York
Albany Madison Avenue Office
879 Madison Ave.
Albany, NY 12208
(518) 438-4150

AIDS Council of Northeastern New York
Glens Falls/Saratoga Office
21 Bay St., Suite 305
Glens Falls, NY 12801
(518) 743-0703

AIDS Council of Northeastern New York
Hudson Office
Fairview Plaza
160 Fairview Ave.
Hudson, NY 12534
(518) 828-3624

AIDS Council of Northeastern New York
Troy Office
313 Tenth St.
Troy, NY 12180
(518) 272-2308

AIDS Council of Northeastern New York
Schenectady Office
434 Franklin St.
Schenectady, NY 12305
(518) 346-9272

AIDS Council of Northeastern New York
Plattsburgh Office
202 Cornelia St., PO Box 903
Plattsburgh, NY 12901
(518) 563-2437, (800) 340-2437

AIDS Community Services of Western New York
206 South Elmwood Ave.
Buffalo, New York 14201
(716) 847-2441

AIDS-Related Community Services (Mid-Hudson Valley)
2269 Saw Mill River Rd., Building 1S
Elmsford, NY 10523
(800) 992-1442

AIDS Center of Queens County
97-45 Queens Blvd., Suite 12th Floor
Rego Park, NY 11374
(718) 896-2500, Ext. 3022

Bronx AIDS Services
1 Fordham Plaza, Suite 903
Bronx, NY 10408
(718) 295-5605

Brooklyn AIDS Task Force
465 Dean St.
Brooklyn, NY 11217
(718) 783-0883

AIDS Rochester
Main Office
1350 University Ave.
Rochester, NY 14607
(585) 442-2220

AIDS Rochester
Geneva Office
605 West Washington St.
Geneva, NY 14456
(315) 781-6303

AIDS Rochester
Bath Office
122 Liberty St.
PO Box 624
Bath, NY 14810
(607) 776-9166

**AIDS Community Resources
of Central New York**
Main Office (Syracuse)
627 West Genesee St.
Syracuse, NY 13204
(315) 475-2430

**AIDS Community Resources
of Central New York**
Utica Office
1119 Elm St.
Utica, NY 13501
(315) 793-0661

**AIDS Community Resources
of Central New York**
Rome Office
212 West Liberty St.
Rome, New York 13440
(315) 336-7523

**AIDS Community Resources
of Central New York**
Watertown Office
165 Mechanic St.
Watertown, NY 13601
(315) 785-8222

**AIDS Community Resources
of Central New York**
Canton Office
7 Main St.
Canton, NY 13617
(315) 386-4493

**AIDS Community Resources
of Central New York**
Auburn Office
27 E. Genesee St.
Auburn, NY 13021
(315) 253-7924, Ext. 34

Southern Tier AIDS Program
Johnson City Location
122 Baldwin St.
Johnson City, NY 13790
(607) 798-1706

Southern Tier AIDS Program
Oneonta Location
31 Main St.
Oneonta, NY 13820
(888) 895-7264

Southern Tier AIDS Program
Elmira Location
330 West Church St.
Elmira, NY 14901
(888) 564-5693

Staten Island AIDS Task Force
42 Richmond Terrace
Staten Island, NY 10301
Hotline: (718) 448-2255
Office: (718) 981-3366

Mother's Voices
165 West 46th St., Suite 701
New York, NY 10036
(212) 730-2777, (888) 686-4237

**Montefiore Medical Center Adolescent
AIDS Program**
35-14 Wayne Ave.
Bronx, NY 10467
(718) 882-0232, (718) 882-0432

Momentum AIDS Project
155 West 23rd St.
New York, NY 10011
(212) 691-8100

**Coalition for the Homeless AIDS
Project**
89 Chambers St.
New York, NY 10007
(212) 964-5900, Ext. 113

**Harlem United Community AIDS
Center**
123-125 West 124th St.
New York, NY 10027
(212) 531-1300

**The Osborne Association AIDS
in Prison Project**
809 Westchester Ave.
Bronx, NY 10455
(718) 842-0500

**New York State Office of AIDS
Discrimination Issues**
(800) 523-2437

Legal Action Center
153 Waverly Pl.
New York, NY 10014
(212) 243-1313

**New York City Gay and Lesbian
Anti-Violence Project**
240 West 35th St., Suite 200
New York, NY 10001
TTY: (212) 714-1134
Bilingual Hotline: (212) 714-1141
(212) 714-1141

National AIDS Treatment Advocacy Project
580 Broadway, Suite 1010
New York, NY 10012
(212) 219-0106, (888) 266-2827

HIV NYC Legal Services
841 Broadway, Suite 608
New York, NY 10003
(212) 674-7590

Tzvi Aryeh AIDS Foundation
PO Box 150
Cathedral Station
New York, NY 10025
(212) 866-6306

Body Positive
19 Fulton St., Suite 308B
New York, NY 10038
(800) 566-6599

Friends in Deed
594 Broadway, Suite 706
New York, NY 10012
(212) 925-2009

Identity House
39 West 14th St., Suite 205
New York, NY 10011
(212) 243-8181

ADAP Plus (Primary Care)
(800) 542-2437

AIDS Drug Assistance Program
(800) 542-2437

AIDS Treatment Data Network
611 Broadway, Suite 613
New York, NY 10012
Hotline: (212) 260-8868
Nationwide: (800) 734-7104

Experimental Treatments Infoline
(800) 633-74448

NORTH CAROLINA
North Carolina AIDS Hotline
In North Carolina: (800) 342-2437
National: (919) 733-3039

AIDS Community Residence Association
PO Box 25265
Durham, NC 27702-5265
(919) 956-7901

Baptist AIDS Partnership of North Carolina
PO Box 1318
Wake Forest, NC 27588-1318
(919) 554-3220

Piedmont HIV Health Care Consortium
Piedmont Consortium
331 West Main St., 5th Floor
Durham, NC 27701
(919) 682-3998, (800) 272-9610

Metrolina AIDS Project (Charlotte)
PO Box 32662
Charlotte, NC 28232
(704) 333-1435

NORTH DAKOTA
North Carolina AIDS Hotline
In North Carolina: (800) 342-2437
National: (919) 733-3039

North Dakota HIV/AIDS Program
600 E. Boulevard Ave.
Bismark, ND 58505
(701) 328-2378

OHIO
Ohio AIDS Hotline
In Ohio: (800) 332-2437
In Ohio TTY/TDD: (800) 332-3889
National: (614) 466-6374

AIDS Resource Center Ohio
211 South Main St., Suite 1000
Dayton, OH 45402
(937) 461-2437

AIDS Taskforce of Greater Cleveland
2728 Euclid Ave., Suite 400
Cleveland, OH 44115-2412
(216) 621-0766 x240

AIDS Volunteers of Cincinnati
220 Findlay St.
Cincinnati, OH 45210
TTD: (513) 421-5030
(513) 421-2437

Caracole
1821 Summit Rd., Suite 001
Cincinnati, OH 45237
(513) 761-1480

The Columbus AIDS Task Force
751 Northwest Blvd.
Columbus, OH 43212-3856
(614) 299-2437

Ohio AIDS Coalition
48 West Whittier St.
Columbus, OH 43206
(614) 444-1683, (800) 226-5554

Project Open Hand-Columbus
82 E 16th Ave.
Columbus, OH 43201
(614) 298-8334

Union County AIDS Task Force
Box 517
Marysville, OH 43040
(937) 642-0801, Ext. 20,
  (888) 333-9461, Ext. 20

OKLAHOMA
Oklahoma AIDS Hotline
In Oklahoma: (800) 535-2437
National: (918) 834-4194

Ahalaya Project/NNAAPC
1211 N. Shartel, Suite 404
Oklahoma City, OK 73103
(405) 235-9988

CarePoint, Consortium of AIDS Resources & Education
1200 North Walker, Suite 500
Oklahoma City, OK 73103
(405) 232-2437
Outside OKC: (800) 285-2273

Oklahoma City Clinic
701 N. E. 10 St.
Oklahoma City, OK 73104
(405) 280-5463

Red Rock Behavioral Health Center
AIDS Counseling Program & Positive Living
  Program
2401 N. W. 39, Suite 100
Oklahoma City, OK
(405) 524-6500

Oklahoma Infant Assistance Program
Child Study Center
1100 N. E. 13 St.
Oklahoma City, OK 73117
(405) 271-6824

Tulsa C.A.R.E.S.
3507 E. Admiral Pl.
Tulsa, OK 74115
(918) 834-4194, (800) 749-4213

OREGON
Oregon AIDS Hotline
Area codes 503, 206, and 208:
  (800) 777-2437
Voice & TTY: (503) 223-2437
National: (503) 223-2437

AIDS Educational Council of Eastern Oregon
PO Box 2901
La Grande, OR 97850
(541) 962-7048, (888) 883-5423

Cascade AIDS Project (Portland)
620 SW Fifth Ave., Suite 300
Portland, OR 97204
(503) 223-5907

Cascade AIDS Project (Clark County)
1104 Main St., Suite M-100
Vancouver, WA 98660
(360) 735-9170

Oregon Public Health Services
800 NE Oregon St.
Portland, OR 97232
(503) 731-4000

Portland Area HIV Services Planning Council
20 NE 10th Ave., 2nd Floor
Portland, OR 97232
(503) 988-3030, Ext. 226

PENNSYLVANIA
Pennsylvania AIDS Hotline
In Pennsylvania: (800) 662-6080
National: (717) 783-0573

ActionAIDS (Central Office)
1216 Arch St., 6th Floor
Philadelphia, PA 19107
(215) 981-0088

ActionAIDS (North Office)
2718 North 5th St.
Philadelphia, PA 19133
(215) 291-9700

Washington West Project
1201 Locust St.
Philadelphia, PA 19107
(215) 985-9206

ActionAIDS (West Office)
3901 Market St.
Philadelphia, PA 19107
(215) 387-6055

**AIDS Service Center in the Greater
Lehigh Valley**
60 W. Broad St., Suite 205
Bethlehem, PA 18018
(610) 974-8700

Berks AIDS Network
PO Box 8626
429 Walnut St.
Reading, PA 19603-8626
(610) 375-6523

Chester County AIDS Support Services
31 South 10th Ave., Suite 2
Coatesville, PA 19320-3561
(610) 466-7848

AIDS Library
1233 Locust St., 2nd Floor
Philadelphia, PA 19107
215-985-4851

Pittsburgh AIDS Task Force
905 West St., Fourth Floor
Pittsburgh, PA 15221
(412) 242-2500

Shepherd Wellness Community
4800 Sciota St.
Pittsburgh, PA 15224
(412) 683-4477

Siloam Ministries
1133 Spring Garden St.
Philadelphia, PA 19123-3315
(215) 765-6633

**Southwestern Pennsylvania AIDS
Planning Coalition**
907 West St., Fifth Floor
Pittsburgh, PA 15221-2841
(412) 242-2441, (877) 732-0401

AIDS Law Project of Pennsylvania
1211 Chestnut St., Suite 600
Philadelphia, PA 19107
(215) 587-9377

AIDS Services in Asian Communities
1201 Chestnut St., 5th Floor
Philadelphia, PA 19107
(215) 563-2424

AIDS Treatment Information Service
1233 Locust St., 5th Floor
Philadelphia, PA 19107
(215) 546-3776

**AIDS Working Groups of Religious
Society of Friends**
1515 Cherry St.
Philadelphia, PA 19102
(215) 241-7238

**Albert Einstein Immunodeficiency
Center**
1335 Tabor Rd., Suite 310
Philadelphia, PA 19141
(215) 224-5623

**BEBASHI (Blacks Educating Blacks
About Sexual Health Issues)**
1217 Spring Garden St.
Philadelphia, PA 19123
(215) 769-3561

Best Nest
1337 Pine St.
Philadelphia, PA 19107
(215) 546-8060

We Care HIV AIDS Support Network
PO Box 1013
Wilkes-Barre, PA 18703-1013
(570) 824-1007

RHODE ISLAND
Rhode Island AIDS Hotline
National: (800) 726-3010

AIDS Care Ocean State
18 Parkis Ave.
Providence, RI 02907
(401) 521-3603

SOUTH CAROLINA
South Carolina AIDS Hotline
In South Carolina: (800) 322-2437
National: (803) 898-0749

AIDS Council of Gaston County
991 West Hudson Blvd.
Gastonia, NC 28053
(704) 853-5101

Catawba Care Coalition
1151 Camden Ave.
Rock Hill, SC 29732
(877) 647-6363

Metrolina AIDS Project
227 East Blvd.
Charlotte, NC 28203
(704) 333-1435, (800) 289-2437

Regional HIV/AIDS Consortium
301 South Brevard St.
Charlotte, NC 28202
(704) 371-6341

SOUTH DAKOTA
South Dakota AIDS Hotline
In South Dakota: (800) 592-1861
National: (605) 773-3737

TENNESSEE
Tennessee AIDS Hotline
In Tennessee: (800) 525-AIDS
National: (615) 741-7500

Chattanooga CARES
PO Box 4497
Chattanooga, TN 37405
(423) 265-2273

Hope Center
1901 Clinch Ave.
Knoxville, TN 37916
(865) 541-3767

Nancy's House
PO Box 5086
Cleveland, TN 37320-5086
(423) 559-8592

Nashville CARES
(800) 845-4266

TEXAS
Texas AIDSLINE
In Texas: (800) 299-2437
National: (572) 490-2500

AIDS Foundation Houston
3202 Weslayan Annex
Houston, TX 77027
(713) 623-6796

AIDS Outreach Center of Tarrant County (Fort Worth)
801 West Cannon
Fort Worth, TX 76104
(817) 335-1994

AIDS Outreach Center of Tarrant County (Arlington)
401 W. Sanford, Suite 1100
Arlington, TX 76011
(817) 275-3311

AIDS Outreach Center of Tarrant County (Southeast)
2516 Oakland Blvd.
Fort Worth, TX 76103
(817) 535-1113

AIDS Resource Center of Dallas
2701 Reagan St.
PO Box 190869
Dallas, TX 75219
(214) 528-0144

AIDS Services of Austin
PO Box 4874
Austin, TX 78765
(512) 458-2437

AIDS Services of North Texas (Denton–Main Office)
4210 Mesa Dr.
Denton, TX 76207
(940) 381-1501, (800) 974-2437

AIDS Services of North Texas (Plano)
1316 14th St.
Plano, TX 75074
(972) 424-1480, (800) 339-2437

AIDS Services of North Texas (Greenville)
3506 Texas St.
Greenville, TX 75401
(903) 450-4018

AIDS Services of North Texas (Rockwall)
Reeves Service Center
102 S. First St.
Rockwall, TX 75087
(800) 974-2437

Alamo Area Resource Center
527 N. Leona
PO Box 7160
San Antonio, TX 78207
(210) 358-9995

Bryan's House
PO Box 35868
Dallas, TX 75235
(214) 559-3946

Center for AIDS in Houston
PO Box 66306
Houston, TX 77266-6306
(713) 527-8219, (888) 341-1788

Montrose Counseling Center
701 Richmond Ave.
Houston, TX 77006
(713) 529-0037

Bering Omega Community Services
PO Box 540517
Houston, TX 77254-0517
(713) 529-6071

Montrose Clinic
215 Westheimer
Houston, TX 77006
(713) 830-3000

San Antonio AIDS Foundation
818 East Grayson
San Antonio, TX 78208-1013
(210) 225-4715

Texas Human Rights Foundation
803 Hawthorne
Houston, TX 77006
(713) 522-0636

UTAH

Utah AIDS Information Line
In Utah: (800) 366-2437
National: (801) 487-2100

Utah AIDS Foundation
1408 South 1100 East
Salt Lake City, UT 84105
(801) 487-2323, (800) 865-5004

VERMONT

Vermont AIDS Hotline
In Vermont: (800) 882-2437
National: (802) 863-7245

New Hampshire/Vermont HIV Information Network
PO Box 882
Bellows Falls, VT 05101
(888) 338-8796

Vermont People With AIDS Coalition
PO Box 11
Montpelier, VT 05601-0011
(802) 229-5754

VIRGINIA

Virginia STD/AIDS Hotline
In Virginia: (800) 533-4148
In Virginia Hispanic line: (800) 322-7432
National: (804) 371-7455

AIDS/HIV Services Group Charlottesville
PO Box 2322
Charlottesville, VA 22902
(804) 979-7714, (800) 752-6862

Central Virginia AIDS Resource and Consultation Center
Box 980147
Richmond, VA 23298-0147
(804) 828-2210, (800) 525-7605

Eastern Regional AIDS Resource and Consultation Center
PO Box 1980
Norfolk, VA 23501-1980
(757) 446-6170

AIDS Response Effort
333 West Cork St.
Winchester, VA 22601
(540) 536-5290

Fredericksburg Area HIV/AIDS Support Services
415 Elm St.
Fredericksburg, VA 22401
(540) 371-7532, (800) 215-8121

Whitman-Walker Clinic of Northern Virginia
(703) 237-4900

Williamsburg AIDS Network
PO Box 1066
Williamsburg, VA 23187-1066
(757) 220-4606

WASHINGTON

Washington AIDS Hotline
In Washington: (800) 272-2437
National: (360) 236-3466

BABES Network
1001 Broadway, Suite 100
Seattle, WA 98122
(206) 720-5566, Ext. 12

Seattle's Bailey-Boushay House
Bailey-Boushay House
2720 East Madison
Seattle, WA 98112
(206) 322-5300

Blue Mountain Heart to Heart
2330 Eastgate St., Suite 105
PO Box 40
Walla Walla, WA 99362
Spanish: (509) 529-2174
(509) 529-4744

Lifelong AIDS Alliance
1002 East Seneca St.
Seattle, WA 98122
(206) 329-6923

Multi-Faith AIDS Project
1801 12th Ave., Suite A
Seattle, WA 98122
(206) 324-1520

North American Syringe Exchange Network
535 Dock St., #1
Tacoma, WA 98402
(253) 272-4857

Pierce County AIDS Foundation
625 Commerce, Suite 10
Tacoma, WA 98402
TTY: (253) 627-7630
(253) 383-2565

Positive Women's Network
3701 Broadway
Everett, WA 98201
(425) 259-9899, (888) 651-8931

Seattle AIDS Support Group
(206) 322-2437

Positive Power
(206) 685-4230

Rise N' Shine
1305 Fourth Ave., Suite 404
Seattle, WA 98101
(206) 628-8949

Seattle Shanti
1801 12th Ave., Suite A
Seattle, WA 98122
(206) 324-1520, Ext. 227

United Communities AIDS Network
1204 East Fourth Ave., Suite 1
Olympia, WA 98506
(360) 352-2375

WEST VIRGINIA

West Virginia AIDS Hotline
In West Virginia: (800) 642-8244
National: (304) 558-2950

AIDS Network
PO Box 2306
Martinsburg, WV 25402
(304) 263-0738, (888) 955-6535

African Americans Want HIV/AIDS Risk Reduction and Education
All-Aid International, Inc.
612 Virginia St. East, Suite 202
Charleston, WV 25301
(304) 343-6202

Tri-State AIDS Task Force
821 4th Ave.
Huntington, WV 25701
(304) 522-4357, (888) 299-2437

Charleston AIDS Network
PO Box 1024
Charleston, WV 25324
(304) 345-4673, (888) 455-4673

Mid-Ohio Valley AIDS Task Force
PO Box 1184
Parkersburg, WV 26102-1184
(304) 485-4803

AIDS Task Force of the Upper Ohio Valley
PO Box 6360
Wheeling, WV 26003
(304) 232-6822

WISCONSIN

Wisconsin AIDS Hotline
In Wisconsin: (800) 334-2437
National: (414) 273-2437

AIDS Resource Center of Wisconsin
Appleton Office
120 North Morrison St., Suite 201
Appleton WI 54911
(920) 733-2068, (800) 773-2068

AIDS Resource Center of Wisconsin
Eau Claire Office
505 Dewey St. South, Suite 107 54701
PO Box 11 54702-0011
Eau Claire, WI
(715) 836-7710, (800) 750-2437

AIDS Resource Center of Wisconsin
Green Bay Office
824 South Broadway
Green Bay WI 54304
(920) 437-7400, (800) 675-9400

AIDS Resource Center of Wisconsin
Kenosha Office
1212 57th St.
Kenosha, WI 53140
PO Box 0173
Kenosha, WI 53141-0173
(262) 657-6644, (800) 924-6601

AIDS Resource Center of Wisconsin
La Crosse Office
Grandview Center 1707
Main St., Suite 420
La Crosse WI 54601
(608) 785-9866, (800) 947-3353

AIDS Resource Center of Wisconsin
Madison Office
222 State St.
Madison WI 53701-0728
(608) 258-9103, (800) 518-9910

AIDS Resource Center of Wisconsin
Milwaukee Office
820 North Plankinton Ave.
PO Box 510498
Milwaukee, WI 53203-0092
(414) 273-1991, (800) 359-9272

AIDS Resource Center of Wisconsin
Superior Office
Board of Trade Building
1507 Tower Ave., Suite 230
Superior, WI 54880
(715) 394-4009, (877) 242-0282

AIDS Resource Center of Wisconsin
Schofield (Wausau) Office
1105 Grand Ave., Suite 3
Schofield, WI 54476
(715) 355-6867, (800) 551-3311

WYOMING
Wyoming AIDS Hotline
National: (800) 327-3577

Puerto Rico
Puerto Rico Linea de Infor SIDA y Enfermedades de Transmision Sexual
In Puerto Rico: (800) 981-5721
National: (809) 765-1010

Puerto Rico Community Network for Clinical Research on AIDS
Brimbaugh Street #1162
Urb. Garci'a Ubarri,
Puerto Rico
(787) 753-9443

Acknowledgments

SEVERAL INDIVIDUALS deserve a nod of apprecia-
tion, not just for assistance in creating this book, but also for
support along the way. I owe my friend and colleague Steve
Baeck many thanks for his encouragement and editorial insight
that helped steer my thinking and this book to a better place.
In addition, several friends deserve acknowledgement: Nancy
Gottesman for supplying real food and for always giving the
right answer to my daily "Am I crazy?" questions; Mark Heins-
sen for returning almost all of my phone calls, almost all of the
time; Joel Moody for graciously handling my antics and crank-
iness; and Diane Baldwin for her photographic skills and for
always lending her ear. I also want to acknowledge my aunt Gail
and my parents, George and Jane, for their love and support.

Keeping me "contained" throughout the writing process was
not easy and so appreciation goes to Monica Farassat for doing
so. Also, Christopher Rowe for holding me together throughout
the dark, early days of the epidemic, Joseph Crump for having
believed in me, and Daniel Berger, M.D., not just for his
involvement in the book, but also for his larger commitment to
advancing health and medicine.

My thanks also goes to Ramon Juarbe at the National Institutes of Health (NIH) for connecting me with the right people;
Anthony Fauci, M.D., also at the NIH, for his time, knowledge,
and contacts; Glenn Gaylord at CorrectHelp for the inside

word; Peg Schumacher, Gregg Pazak, and many colleagues at RAND for their understanding and flexibility; Richard Klein at the Food and Drug Administration for good advice; and Baruch Fischhoff at Carnegie Mellon University for insights and edits.

On the publishing side, my appreciation goes to Marlowe & Company's Suzanne McCloskey, whose skillful editing, patience, and hands-on problem solving made this book possible and my experience enjoyable; Matthew Lore for creating the First Year series, William Finley Green for referring me to Matthew; Howard Grossman for cover design; and Pauline Neuwirth for interior page design.

Finally, my deepest gratitude extends to all of the individuals cited throughout these pages for their trust, life lessons, and strength of character to speak out despite the stigma, fear, and consequences that still come with being honest about HIV and AIDS.

Index

A

abacavir (Ziagen), 231,
242–43
ACE inhibitors, 138, 267
activism, 263
Act Up New York, 263
acupuncture, 82
acute infection, 32, 63, 267
acyclovir, 110–11
ADA (Americans with Dis-
abilities Act), 187–96
ADAP (AIDS Drug Assis-
tance Programs), 179–80
addiction
See also substance abuse
determining if you have
an, 143
fixing, 142–50
sex, 149–50
treatment
detox is not, 144
double-action, 144–45
effective, 145–46
facilities for, 142–43
medications for,
146–47
options in, 147–49
self-help groups for,
148–49
twelve-step programs,
148–49
adefovir (Hepsera), 219, 222
adherence, 208, 234–37,
246–47

agonist maintenance treatment, 146
AIDS
activism, 263
immune system and,
48–49
is caused by HIV, 15
myth, 73–74
opportunistic infections
of, 168
transmission of, 21
vaccines, 32
vs. HIV, 2, 31–32, 72–73
AIDS Action, 263
AIDS cocktail, 64, 206, 212,
220
AIDS Drug Assistance Pro-
grams (ADAP), 179–80
AIDS InfoNet.Org, 264
AIDS service organizations
finding, 35
health insurance and,
176–78
services offered by, 12,
28–30, 175–76
AIDS wasting, 152, 231–33
alcohol, 135–36, 216
Alcoholics Anonymous (AA),
148–49
allergic reactions, 242–43
alternative medicine
effectiveness of, 33,
77–78
for the mind, 81–83

popularity of, 76–77
Americans with Disabilities
Act (ADA), 187–96
amphetamines, 138–39, 267
anal cancer, 113
anal sex, 99, 101–3, 115
anger, 9–10
angiotensin converting
enzyme (ACE) inhibitors,
138, 267
anilingus, 99, 267
Antabuse, 147
antagonist treatment, 146
anti-AIDS cults, 74–75
anti-anxiety drugs, 5, 130–31
antibodies, 62
antidepressants, 129–30
antiretrovirals, 63, 267
antivirals, 63–64, 267
anxiety
about, 118–19
as reaction to diagnosis,
4–6
treatment for, 124–31
aspartate transaminase
(AST), 221, 267
aspergillosis, 136, 267
asymptomatic shedding, 109,
268
atazanavir (Reyataz), 212
AZT (Retrovir), 231

B

barebacking, 102–3, 268

Bartlett, John G., 217
bDNA, 87, 171, 268
benzodiazepines, 131, 137, 268
Berger, Daniel, 7, 79–81, 245, 247, 249–51, 254
blame
    of God, 25–26
    self, 8–9
blood sugar abnormalities, 226–27
blood tests
    HIV viral load, 41, 84–89, 171–73
    initial, 59–60
    T-cell counts, 41, 60, 84–89, 170–71
    tracking, in health journal, 40–41
body shape changes
    combating, 230–33
    reasons for, 228–29
    as side effect, 227–28
brain, drug use and, 133–34
Brewi, Timothy M., 163
buprenorphine, 146–47
buspirone (BuSpar), 131, 268

C
cancer, 112–13, 115
candidiasis, 268
cardio exercise, 162–63, 229
Cava, Edmund, 4
CD4+ cell, 62–63, 268
    See also T-cell counts
cervical cancer, 113, 115
children, having, 256–60
chiropractic care, 82
cholesterol, 41, 227–28
cigarettes, 135, 143–44
clinical social workers, 127
clinical trials, 181
COBRA, 178
cocaine, 137–38
co-infection
    with genital warts, 106–7, 112–15
    with hepatitis B, 219–20
    with hepatitis C, 215–18
    with herpes, 106–12
Coles, Matthew, 187
combination therapy, 64, 206, 212, 220
Community Reinforcement Approach, 147–48
compliance, 208
    See also adherence

compulsion, 149
condoms, 100–1, 103–5
counselors, 127
co-workers, disclosing HIV status to, 69
crack, 137–38
crying, 4
crystal meth, 138–39
cunnilingus, 98–99, 268

D
dating, 93–95
    See also sex
denial, 7–8, 27, 166–67
dental care, 18–19, 29
dental dams, 99, 268
dentists, disclosing HIV status to, 67
depression
    about, 120–22
    in people with HIV, 59
    treatment for, 124–31
detox, 144
diabetes mellitus, 155, 226, 268
diacetylmorphine (heroin), 140, 268
diagnosis
    adjusting to, 47–49
    reaction to, 1–10, 117–18
    telling others about, 11–13, 65–70
    tips for coping with, 5
diarrhea, 239, 241–42
diet, healthy, 156–58, 231
dietary supplements, 78–81, 125–26, 158
Disability Determination Service (DDS), 183
disassociation, 7, 268
disclosure
    being selective about, 11–13
    dating and, 93–95
    pros and cons of, 65–70
    tactics, 95
discrimination
    ADA (Americans with Disabilities Act) and, 187–96
    health insurance, 194
    protection from, 13
    reasonable accommodations and, 190–91
    recognizing, 188–89
    safety issues and, 191–93
    by state and local governments, 194–95

taking action against, 194–96
    workplace, 186–96
DNA, 87, 268
doctors
    disclosing HIV status to, 67
    finding good HIV, 53–60
    honesty with, 246–48
    initial visit with, 58–60
    relationships with, 57–58
    trusting, 33
dopamine, 134, 149
drug holidays, 209
drug-naïve, 207
drugs
    See also addiction; substance abuse; treatment
    ADAP (AIDS Drug Assistance Programs) for, 179–80
    for addiction treatment, 146–47
    adefovir (Hepsera), 21, 222
    adherence to, 208, 234–37, 246–47
    advances in, xii, 2, 214
    allergic reactions to, 242–43
    anti-anxiety, 5, 130–31
    antidepressants, 129–30
    antivirals, 63–64, 267
    combination therapy, 64, 206, 212, 220
    fusion inhibitors, 213, 254–55
    for hepatitis, 219–20, 222
    lamivudine (Epivir), 219, 222
    for mood disorders, 129–31
    non-nucleoside reverse transcriptase inhibitors (non-nukes), 213, 228
    nucleoside reverse transcriptase inhibitors (nukes), 211–12, 228
    once-a-day dosing of, 208–9
    protease inhibitors (PIs), xii, 155, 212–14, 226–28, 269
    reasons for, 2, 134–35
    recreational, 132–41
    resistance to, 206–7, 249, 254
    side effects from, 225–29, 238–43

tenofovir (Viread), 212, 219–20, 222
tracking, in health journal, 42
Duesberg, Peter, 73–74
dysplasia, 112–13, 115, 268

E
Echinacea, 79–80
Ecstasy, 140, 268
efavirenz (Sustiva), 213
emotions
  about sex, 95–96
  after initial diagnosis, 4–10, 117–18
  anger, 9–10
  anxiety, 4–6, 118–19
  depression, 59, 120–22
  sadness, 120
  self-blame, 8–9
  shame, 21–22
  talking about your, 8
employment discrimination, 186–96
emtricitabine, 222
enfuvirtide (Fuzeon), 213, 254–55
Epivir (lamivudine), 219, 222
exercise
  benefits of, 5, 125, 160, 229, 231
  inner fat and, 161, 231
  strength training, 163–65
  target zone for, 162
  tracking, in health journal, 40

F
faith, 24–27
famciclovir, 111
family, disclosing HIV status to, 11–12, 69
Famvir, 111
FAQs, 31–33
fat, inner, 161, 231
fatigue, 242
Fauci, Anthony, 18, 32, 54, 136, 156, 161, 200–3, 210, 214, 216, 219–20, 261
fears, 8
feelings. See emotions
fever, 239
friends, disclosing HIV status to, 67
fruits, 158
Fung, John, 224

fusion inhibitors, 213, 254–55
Fuzeon (enfuvirtide), 213, 254–55

G
garlic supplements, 80
generalized anxiety disorder, 118
genes, addiction and, 133
genital herpes. See herpes
genital warts
  cause of, 112
  defined, 268
  HIV and, 106–7, 112–13
  symptoms of, 113
  transmission, 113–14
  treatment, 114–15
genotypic tests, 251, 254, 268
glucose, 226, 268
goals, recording, 42–43
God
  blaming, 25–26
  faith in, as healing power, 24–25
group therapy, 126

H
HAART (highly active anti-retroviral therapy), 64, 268
HDL (high-density lipoprotein), 227–28
headaches, 240–41
HEAL (Health Education AIDS Liaison), 74–75
healthcare
  See also doctors
  access to, 175–85
  managed care, 58
  through clinical trials, 181
Health Education AIDS Liaison (HEAL), 74–75
health history, 58–59
health insurance
  ADAP (AIDS Drug Assistance Programs) and, 179–80
  AIDS organizations and, 176–78
  choosing doctor and, 55–56
  COBRA, 178
  employment discrimination and, 194
  high-risk, 179
  Medicaid, 182

Medical Information Bureau (MIB) and, 178–79
Social Security disability insurance (SSDI), 182
Health Insurance Portability and Accountability Act (HIPAA), 177
health journals
  example of, 44
  purpose of, 39–40
  setting up, 43
  tracking details in, 40–43, 184
healthy thinking, 17–19
heart problems, 138, 228
heart rate, 162
hepatitis
  hepatitis A, 216
  hepatitis B (HBV), 216, 219–20
  hepatitis C (HCV), 215–18
  treating, 221–24
Hepsera (adefovir), 219, 222
herbal medicine, 78–81, 125–26
Herek, Gregory M., 21
heroin, 140, 268
herpes
  about, 107
  HIV and, 106, 110
  prevalence of, 107
  symptoms of, 108–9
  tests for, 110–11
  tracking, in health journal, 41
  transmission, 109–10
  treatments, 111–12
HGH (human growth hormone), 231–33
high-density lipoprotein (HDL), 227–28
Hirschel, Bernard, 202
HIV
  See also HIV-positive
  and AIDS, 2, 15, 31–32, 72–73
  controlled vs. uncontrolled, 153–54, 156
  diabetes and, 155
  effects of, on health, xi–xii
  facts about, 14–16
  future for, 261
  genital warts and, 112–13
  hepatitis and, 215–24
  herpes and, 110

information sources, 262, 264–65
is manageable condition, 1
is not a punishment, 15–16
myths about, 71–74
organ transplants and, 224
origins of, 14–15
resistant strains of, 207, 235–36, 249, 251
substance abuse and, 132–33
symptoms of, 32
transmission, 15, 20–21, 96–103, 257–58
treatment. *See* treatment
workings of, 61–62, 63
HIVandHepatitis.com, 265
HIV-positive
disclosing status of, 11–13, 65–70, 93–95
having children while, 256–60
initial response to, 1–10
lifestyle and, 2–3
need for medicine and, 2
overweight and, 151–53
psychological impact of, 119
reactions from others to, 1, 11–13
shame of, 21–22
stigma of, 20–21, 27
HIV viral load. *See* viral load
HPV (human papillo-mavirus). *See* genital warts
HSV. *See* herpes
human growth hormone (HGH), 231–33
human papillomavirus (HPV). *See* genital warts
hypochondria, 39, 43, 45–46, 269

I
immune system
boosting your, 79
diet and, 153–54, 156
hepatitis B virus (HBV) and, 219
reaction of, to HIV, 62–64
strength of your, 48–49, 88–89
T-cells and, 85–86
infertility, 259
information sources, 262, 264–65
insulin resistance, 226–27

interferon, 222
interindividual variability, 209, 240
intra-abdominal fat, 161, 231
in vitro fertilization, 258–59

J
Jonker, Jelka, 5, 8, 21, 175–76, 258, 262

K
kaposi's sarcoma, 246, 269
kava, 126
Keye, William, Jr., 259
Koenig, Harold, 25
Kramer, Larry, 224

L
lamivudine (Epivir), 219, 222
LDL (low-density lipopro-tein), 227–28
Leshner, Alan, 133–35
Levin, Jules, 219
lifestyle, active, 2–3
lipid abnormalities, 227–28
lipodystrophy, 152, 159, 227–28, 269
lipohypertrophy, 228, 269
liver
biopsies, 223
damage, 221
disease, 217–19
tests (AST), 41
transplants, 224
log, 269
low-density lipoprotein (LDL), 227–28

M
managed care, 58
MAOIs (monoamine oxidase inhibitors), 129, 269
marijuana, 136
massage, 82
masturbation, 96–97
Medicaid, 182
medical care
See also doctors; treatment
religious beliefs conflict-ing with, 26–27
Medical Information Bureau (MIB), 178–79
medical tests
for herpes, 110–11
HIV viral load, 41, 84–89, 171–73

initial, 59–60
T-cell counts, 41, 60, 84–89, 170–71
medications. *See* drugs
meditation, 82, 125
Mediterranean Diet, 156–57, 228
mental health professionals, 127–29
methadone maintenance pro-grams, 147
methamphetamine (crystal meth), 138–39, 269
methylenedioxymethamphet-amine (MDMA), 140, 269
monoamine oxidase inhibitors (MAOIs), 129, 269
mood shifts, tracking, 41–42
morphine, 140
Munk, Bob, 27, 208, 209–10, 212, 214, 218, 246, 247–48, 250
myths, 71–74

N
NATAP.org, 265
nausea, 238–39, 241
needle-exchange programs, 36–37
needles, 36–38, 141
negative thinking, 41–42
Nelson, Mark, 215–16
nevirapine (Viramune), 213, 243
nicotine replacement ther-apy, 143–44
non-nucleoside reverse tran-scriptase inhibitors (non-nukes), 213, 228
nonoxynol-9 (N-9), 100, 269
Norvir (ritonavir), 139, 228
nucleoside reverse transcrip-tase inhibitors (nukes), 211–12, 228
nutrition
basics, 152–53, 156–58
HIV and, 153–54, 156
tracking, in health journal, 40
nutritional problems, xii–xiii

O
obesity, 151–53
obsessive-compulsive behav-ior, 149–50
once-a-day dosing, 208–9
one-night stands, 68–69

opportunistic infections, xii,
15, 168, 269
oral health care, 18–19, 29
oral herpes, 107, 109
oral sex, 98–99
organ transplants, 224
outpatient treatment, 147
overweight, 151–53

P

panic disorder, 119
Pap smears, 115
parents, disclosing HIV status to, 69–70
partial serotonin reuptake
inhibitors, 130, 269
partner, disclosing HIV status to, 66–67
pathogenesis, 63, 269
PCR, 87, 171, 269
pharmaceutical companies, 33
phenotypic tests, 251, 269
physician assisted suicide,
123
physicians. *See* doctors
phytochemicals, 158
pill burden, 212, 269
pneumocystis carinii pneumonia (PCP), 269
Positively Aware (magazine),
264
post-traumatic stress disorder, 119
Poz (magazine), 264
pregnancy, 257–58
priorities, 42–43
prodrome, 108, 269
protease inhibitors (PIs)
about, 212–13
advances in, 214
defined, 269
diabetes and, 155
side effects from, 226–28
as treatment option, xii
psychiatrists, 127
psychologists, 68, 127
psychotherapy, 126–29, 269
Purple Coneflower (Echi-
nacea), 79–80

Q

Qi, 269

R

rashes, 239
recreational substances. *See*
addiction; drugs, recre-
ational; substance abuse

relationships
doctor-patient, 57–58
romantic, 93–95
therapist-patient, 128–29
religion, 23–27
residential programs, 147
resistance, 206–7, 249, 254
resistance testing, 251, 254
resistance training, 163–65,
229
resistant virus, 207, 235–36,
249, 251
resources, 273–98
Retrovir (AZT), 231
retrovirus, 63, 269
Reyataz (atazanavir), 212
ribavirin, 222
rimming, 99
risky behavior, 31
ritonovir (Norvir), 139, 228
RNA, 87, 269

S

sadness, 120
safe sex, 35, 96–97
Safren, Steven A., 15
salvage therapy, 254, 270
Schacker, Timothy, 110
sedatives, 5, 137, 270
self-blame, 8–9
self-help groups, 148–49
semen, 97
sequencing, 207–8
Serostim, 231–33
serotonin, 122, 270
serotonin reuptake inhibitors
(SSRIs), 130
services
free, 28–30
offered by AIDS organiza-
tions, 28–30, 175–76
sex
anal, 99, 101–3, 115
emotions about, 95–96
HIV diagnosis's effect on,
33
masturbation, 96–97
oral, 98–99
safe, 35, 96–97
transmission of HIV and,
96–103
vaginal, 100–1
sex addiction, 149–50
sex partners, disclosing HIV
status to, 68–69
sexually transmitted disease
(STDs)
condom use to prevent, 103

defined, 270
genital warts, 106–7,
112–15
herpes, 106–12
sexual practices, questions
about, 59
shame, 21–22
siblings, disclosing HIV status to, 69
side effects
allergic reactions, 242–43
blood sugar abnormalities,
226–27
body shape changes,
227–33
diarrhea, 239, 241–42
fatigue, 242
fever, 239
headaches, 240–41
insulin resistance, 226–27
lipid abnormalities,
227–28
long-term, 42, 203,
225–29
nausea, 238–39, 241
rash, 239
short-term, 238–43
tracking, in health journal,
42
variations in, 239
vomiting, 241
smoking, 135, 143–44
Social Security benefits,
181–85
defining disability for,
182–85
Medicaid, 182
Social Security disability
insurance (SSDI), 182
Supplemental Security
Income (SSI), 182
Social Security disability
insurance (SSDI), 182
spirituality, 23–27
spouse/partner, disclosing
HIV status to, 66–67
SSRIs (serotonin reuptake
inhibitors), 130
St. John's Wort, 80, 125–26
stavudine (Zerit), 211, 231
stigma, 20–21, 27
strength training, 163–65,
229
structured treatment interruptions, 209
substance abuse, 132–41
See also addiction
of alcohol, 135–36

of amphetamines, 138–39
of benzodiazepines, 137
brain and, 133–34
of cocaine, 137–38
of crystal meth, 138–39
of Ecstasy, 140
genetic tendency toward,
133
of heroin, 140
HIV and, 132–33
of marijuana, 136
needles and, 36–38, 141
reasons for, 134–35
of tobacco, 135
suicidal thoughts, 116–17,
122–23
Supplemental Security
Income (SSI), 182
supplements, 78–81,
125–26, 158
support groups, 34–35
Survive AIDS, 263
Sustiva (efavirenz), 213
symptoms, 32

T
talk therapy, 126–29
Tapia, John, 232
T-cell counts
meaning of, 63
ranges of, 170–71
starting treatment and,
200–1
testing, 41, 60, 84–89
T-cells, 62, 270
tenofovir (Viread), 212,
219–20, 222
testosterone, 231
tests. See medical tests
tetrahydrocannabinol (THC),
136, 270
therapeutic communities,
147
therapists
disclosing HIV status to,
68
finding, 127–29
therapy, 126–29
thrush, 268
topical creams, for herpes,
111
tranquilizers, 137
transmission
of genital warts, 113–14

of herpes, 109–10
of HIV, 15, 20–21, 97
during pregnancy, 257–58
through sexual contact,
96–103
treatment
See also drugs
adherence to, 208,
234–37, 246–47
advances in, xii, 209–10,
249–50
for AIDS wasting, 231–33
antivirals, 63–64
for anxiety, 124–31
for body shape changes,
231–33
case study, 252–53
combination therapy, 64,
206, 212, 220
deciding to start/delay,
47–48
decisions about, 167, 169,
199–205, 210
delaying, 173
for depression, 124–31
expectations, 250
failure, 249–55
future for, 261
for genital warts, 114–15
goals of, 169
guidelines, 169
for hepatitis, 221–24
for herpes, 111–12
interruptions, 250–51
key considerations in,
206–9
long-term effects of, 42,
203, 225–29
rising viral load during,
244–48
second-line, 250, 254–55
side effects from, 42, 203,
225–29, 238–43
starting, 173–74, 204–5
strategies, 199–205
success of, 202–3
T-cell counts and, 170–71
viral load and, 171–73
vs. denial, 166–67
treatment-naïve, 207
tricyclics, 129, 270
triglycerides, 41, 227–28
twelve-step programs,
148–49

U
urban legends, 71–72
urine, 99

V
vaccination records, 41
vaccines, 32, 216
vaginal sex, 100–1
valacyclovir, 111
Valium, 137
Valtrex, 111
vegetables, 158
viral hepatitis. See hepatitis
viral load
defined, 270
progression of disease
and, 171–73
rising, 244–48
starting treatment and,
201
testing, 41, 60, 62–63,
84–89
viral resistance, 206–7,
249
Viramune (nevirapine),
213, 243
Viread (tenofovir), 212,
219–20, 222
vitamin supplements, 158
vomiting, 241

W
warts. See genital warts
wasting, 152, 231–33
Web sites, 264–65
weight lifting, 163–65,
229
Whiteley Index, 43, 45–46
workplace discrimination,
186–96

X
Xanax, 137

Y
yeast infections, 268
yoga, 81, 125

Z
Zerit (stavudine), 211,
231
Ziagen (abacavir), 231,
242–43
Zovirax, 111